CARDIOLOGY RESEARCH AND CLINICAL DEVELOPMENTS SERIES

ABDOMINAL AORTIC ANEURYSMS: NEW APPROACHES TO RUPTURE RISK ASSESSMENT

CARDIOLOGY RESEARCH AND CLINICAL DEVELOPMENTS SERIES

Focus on Atherosclerosis Research
Leon V. Clark (Editor)
2004. ISBN: 1-59454-044-6

Cholesterol in Atherosclerosis and Coronary Heart Disease
Jean P. Kovala (Editor)
2005. ISBN: 1-59454-302-X

Frontiers in Atherosclerosis Research
Karin F. Kepper (Editor)
2007. ISBN: 1-60021-371-5

Cardiac Arrhythmia Research Advances
Lynn A. Vespry (Editor)
2007. ISBN: 1-60021-794-X

Cardiac Arrhythmia Research Advances
Lynn A. Vespry (Editor)
2007. ISBN: 978-1-60692-539-3
(Online Book)

Heart Disease in Women
Benjamin V. Lardner and
Harrison R. Pennelton (Editors)
2009. ISBN: 978-1-60692-066-4

Heart Disease in Women
Benjamin V. Lardner and
Harrison R. Pennelton (Editors)
2010. ISBN: 978-1-60741-090-4
(Online Book)

Cardiomyopathies: Causes, Effects and Treatment
Peter H. Bruno and
Matthew T. Giordano (Editors)
2009. ISBN: 978-1-60692-193-7

Cardiomyopathies: Causes, Effects and Treatment
Peter H. Bruno and
Matthew T. Giordano (Editors)
2009. ISBN: 978-1-60876-433-4
(Online Book)

Transcatheter Coil Embolization of Visceral Arterial Aneurysms
Shigeo Takebayashi, Izumi Torimoto
and Kiyotaka Imoto (Editors)
2009. ISBN: 978-1-60741-439-1

Transcatheter Coil Embolization of Visceral Arterial Aneurysms
Shigeo Takebayashi, Izumi Torimoto
and Kiyotaka Imoto (Editors)
2009. ISBN: 978-1-60876-797-7
(Online Book)

Heart Disease in Men
*Alice B. Todd and
Margo H. Mosley (Editors)*
2009. ISBN: 978-1-60692-297-2

**Angina Pectoris: Etiology,
Pathogenesis and Treatment**
*Alice P. Gallos and
Margaret L. Jones (Editors)*
2009. ISBN: 978-1-60456-674-1

Coronary Artery Bypasses
*Russell T. Hammond and
James B Alton (Editors)*
2009. ISBN: 978-1-60741-064-5

**Congenital Heart Defects: Etiology,
Diagnosis and Treatment**
Hiroto Nakamura (Editor)
2009. ISBN: 978-1-60692-559-1

**Congenital Heart Defects: Etiology,
Diagnosis and Treatment**
Hiroto Nakamura (Editor)
2009. ISBN: 978-1-60876-434-1
(Online Book))

**Atherosclerosis: Understanding
Pathogenesis and Challenge for
Treatment**
*Slavica Mitrovska,
Silvana Jovanova Inge Matthiesen
and Christian Libermans*
2009. ISBN: 978-1-60692-677-2

**Practical Rapid ECG
Interpretation (PREI)**
*Abraham G. Kocheril
and Ali A. Sovari*
2009. ISBN: 978-1-60741-021-8

**Heart Transplantation: Indications
and Contraindications,
Procedures and Complications**
Catherine T. Fleming (Editor)
2009. ISBN 978-1-60741-228-1

**Handbook of Cardiovascular
Research**
Jorgen Brataas and Viggo Nanstveit
2009. ISBN: 978-1-60741-792-7

**Estrogen and Myocardial
Infarction**
*Jiang Hong, Chen Jing,
He Bo, and Lu Zhi-bing*
2010. ISBN: 978-1-60692-257-6

**Advances in Cardiovascular
Research, Volume 1**
*Lukas Schmitt and Timm König
(Editors)*
2010. ISBN: 978-1-60741-720-0

**Heart Transplantation: Indications
and Contraindications,
Procedures and Complications**
Catherine T. Fleming (Editor)
2010. ISBN 978-1-60876-591-1
(Online Book)

Heart Disease in Children
*Marius D. Oliveira and
William S. Copley (Editors)*
2009. ISBN: 978-1-60741-504-6

Heart Disease in Children
*Marius D. Oliveira and
William S. Copley (Editors)*
2009. ISBN: 978-1-61668-225-5
(Online Book)

Handbook of Cardiovascular Research
*Jorgen Brataas
and Viggo Nanstveit (Editors)*
2009. ISBN: 978-1-60741-792-7

Comprehensive Models of Cardiovascular and Respiratory Systems: Their Mechanical Support and Interactions
*Marek Darowski and
Gianfranco Ferrari (Editors)*
2009. ISBN: 978-1-60876-212-5

Cardiac Rehabilitation
Jonathon T. Halliday (Editor)
2010. ISBN: 978-1-60741-918-1

**Cardiovascular Signals in Diabetes Mellitus:
A New Tool to Detect Autonomic Neuropathy**
*Michal Javorka, Ingrid Tonhajzerova,
Zuzana Turianikova,
Kamil Javorka, Natasa Honzikova
and Mathias Baumert*
2010. ISBN: 978-1-60876-788-5

Oxidative Stress: A Focus on Cardiovascular Disease Pathogensis
*Bashir M. Matata
and Maqsood M. Elahi*
2010. ISBN: 978-1-61668-157-9

Oxidative Stress: A Focus on Cardiovascular Disease Pathogensis
*Bashir M. Matata
and Maqsood M. Elahi*
2010. ISBN: 978-1-61668-359-7

Treatment of Ventricular Fibrillation
*Rajiv Sankaranarayanan,
Hanney Gonna, and Michael James*
2010. ISBN: 978-1-60876-850-9

Cardiac Rehabilitation in Women
Arzu Daşkapan
2010. ISBN: 978-1-61668-146-3

Cardiac Rehabilitation in Women
Arzu Daşkapan
2010. ISBN: 978-1-61668-398-6

Abdominal Aortic Aneurysms: New Approaches to Rupture Risk Assessment
*Barry J. Doyle, David S. Molony,
Michael T. Walsh
and Timothy M. McGloughlin*
2010. ISBN: 978-1-61668-312-2

**Biophysical Principles
of Hemodynamics**
*A. N. Volobuev, V. I. Koshev.,
and E.S. Petrov*
2010. ISBN: 978-1-61668-280-4

**Congestive Heart Failure:
Symptoms, Causes and
Treatment**
*Josias E. García
and Victoro R. Wright (Editors)*
2010. ISBN: 978-1-60876-677-2

**Resuscitation of Patients
in Ventricular Fibrillation
from the Perspective of
Emergency Medical Services**
*Paul W. Baker
and Hugh J.M. Grantham*
2010. ISBN: 978-1-60876-668-0

**Myocardial Ischemia: Causes,
Symptoms and Treatment**
*Dmitry Vukovic
and Vladimir Kiyan (Editors)*
2010. ISBN: 978-1-60876-610-9

CARDIOLOGY RESEARCH AND CLINICAL DEVELOPMENTS SERIES

ABDOMINAL AORTIC ANEURYSMS: NEW APPROACHES TO RUPTURE RISK ASSESSMENT

BARRY J. DOYLE,
DAVID S. MOLONY
MICHAEL T. WALSH
AND
TIMOTHY M. MCGLOUGHLIN
EDITORS

Nova Science Publishers, Inc.
New York

Copyright © 2010 by Nova Science Publishers, Inc.

All rights reserved. No part of this book may be reproduced, stored in a retrieval system or transmitted in any form or by any means: electronic, electrostatic, magnetic, tape, mechanical photocopying, recording or otherwise without the written permission of the Publisher.

For permission to use material from this book please contact us:
Telephone 631-231-7269; Fax 631-231-8175
Web Site: http://www.novapublishers.com

NOTICE TO THE READER

The Publisher has taken reasonable care in the preparation of this book, but makes no expressed or implied warranty of any kind and assumes no responsibility for any errors or omissions. No liability is assumed for incidental or consequential damages in connection with or arising out of information contained in this book. The Publisher shall not be liable for any special, consequential, or exemplary damages resulting, in whole or in part, from the readers' use of, or reliance upon, this material.

Independent verification should be sought for any data, advice or recommendations contained in this book. In addition, no responsibility is assumed by the publisher for any injury and/or damage to persons or property arising from any methods, products, instructions, ideas or otherwise contained in this publication.

This publication is designed to provide accurate and authoritative information with regard to the subject matter covered herein. It is sold with the clear understanding that the Publisher is not engaged in rendering legal or any other professional services. If legal or any other expert assistance is required, the services of a competent person should be sought. FROM A DECLARATION OF PARTICIPANTS JOINTLY ADOPTED BY A COMMITTEE OF THE AMERICAN BAR ASSOCIATION AND A COMMITTEE OF PUBLISHERS.

LIBRARY OF CONGRESS CATALOGING-IN-PUBLICATION DATA

```
3D imaging of abdominal aortic aneurysms : techniques and applications
/ Barry J. Doyle ... [et al.].
       p. ; cm.
   Includes index.
   ISBN 978-1-61668-312-2 (softcover)
   1.  Abdominal aneurysm--Imaging. 2.  Three-dimensional imaging in
medicine.  I. Doyle, Barry J.
   [DNLM: 1.  Aortic Aneurysm, Abdominal--diagnosis. 2.  Imaging,
Three-Dimensional--methods.  WG 410 Z3 2010]
   RC693.A14 2010
   616.1'330754--dc22
                                                     2010001053
```

Published by Nova Science Publishers, Inc. † New York

Contents

Preface		xi
Chapter 1	Introduction	1
Chapter 2	3D Reconstruction from CT Scans	9
Chapter 3	Applications of AAA 3D Reconstructions	13
Chapter 4	Numerical Investigations	15
Chapter 5	Experimental Investigations	43
Chapter 6	Conclusion	63
Acknowledgments		65
References		67
Index		77

PREFACE

BACKGROUND

The advancements in medical imaging technology over the last number of years has revolutionised the management and treatment of all aspects of healthcare. Computed tomography and magnetic resonance imaging have led to the development of reconstruction software that allows internal bodily structures to be easily visualised in 3D. These developments have led to improved surgical planning and treatment. The assessment of abdominal aortic aneurysms (AAA) has benefited greatly from these advancements. There is currently much debate as when to surgically repair these life-threatening dilations of the aorta and 3D reconstructions of AAAs have led to many new diagnostic tools and rupture-prediction indices. This chapter explores some of the more recent developments in this area.

METHODS

Imaging of patient-specific AAAs opens many possibilities for the surgical-planning and biomechanical examination of the diseased vessel. 3D reconstructions allow for exact measurements and dimensions of stent-grafts to be obtained. These 3D reconstructions also form the basis for all numerical modelling techniques, be it finite element analysis, computational fluid dynamics or fluid-structure interaction. Computational and experimental examination of the wall stress within a particular AAA can reveal important information regarding possible rupture sites, and relationships between wall stress and geometrical factors. 3D imaging has allowed the development of new parameters that may better assess the likelihood of AAA rupture on a patient-specific basis. Post-operative monitoring of the stent-graft also benefits from 3D imaging. The *in-vivo* pulsatile forces acting on the stent-graft, which contribute to stent-graft migration and may result in sac re-pressurisation, can be numerically determined on a patient-specific basis. The use of 3D reconstructions also allows for improved experimental testing through exact AAA replications and numerical validation models.

RESULTS

New diagnostic tools and rupture-prediction methods have revealed that similarly sized AAAs may have significantly different rupture potentials. Experimental approaches to AAA assessment have shown that AAAs will rupture at regions of elevated wall stress and not at areas of maximum diameter. Fluid-structure interaction is a useful tool for assessing post-operative stent-graft performance, as both the haemodynamic forces acting on the stent-graft and wall stress of the aneurysm are of interest. Numerical modelling has also allowed for the design and evaluation of novel stent-graft designs such as the tapered device presented in this chapter.

CONCLUSION

3D imaging has allowed engineers to aid clinicians in the management and treatment of AAAs. 3D reconstructions form the basis for many engineering techniques, both numerical and experimental, and help contribute to the decision to either surgically intervene and repair an AAA, or monitor the expansion of the AAA with regular imaging. There is a need to implement alternative factors in the clinical decision-making process and the methodologies reported in this chapter may be beneficial in future AAA rupture assessment and management.

Chapter 1

INTRODUCTION

1.1. INCIDENCE AND CURRENT OPINIONS

Cardiovascular disease is the leading cause of morbidity and premature death of modern era medicine. It is estimated that approximately 81 million people in the United States (US) currently have one or more of the many forms of cardiovascular disease, resulting in 1 in every 2.8 deaths, or 900,000 deaths per year. 40% of all deaths in Europe are a result of cardiovascular disease in people under the age of 75, with mortality rates in Ireland reported to be as high as 43% in 1997 [Creagh et al., 2002]. Aneurysms form a significant portion of these cardiovascular related deaths and are defined as a permanent and irreversible localised dilation of a blood vessel greater than 50% of its normal diameter [Sakalihasan et al., 2005]. Although aneurysms can form in any blood vessel, the more lethal aneurysms develop in the cranial arteries, thoracic aorta and abdominal aorta, which if left untreated, will eventually expand until rupture. The vast majority of these aneurysms form in the abdominal aorta and are termed abdominal aortic aneurysm (AAA). Figure 1 shows a comparison between a healthy young male and the diseased aorta of an elderly male patient. The actual mechanisms resulting in AAA formation are still not fully understood. It is believed that these aneurysms form due to alterations of the connective tissue in the aortic wall. The degradation of the aortic wall can be attributed to risk factors such as tobacco smoking, gender, age, hypertension, chronic obstructive pulmonary disease, hyperlipidaemia and family history of the disorder [Sakalihasan et al., 2005].

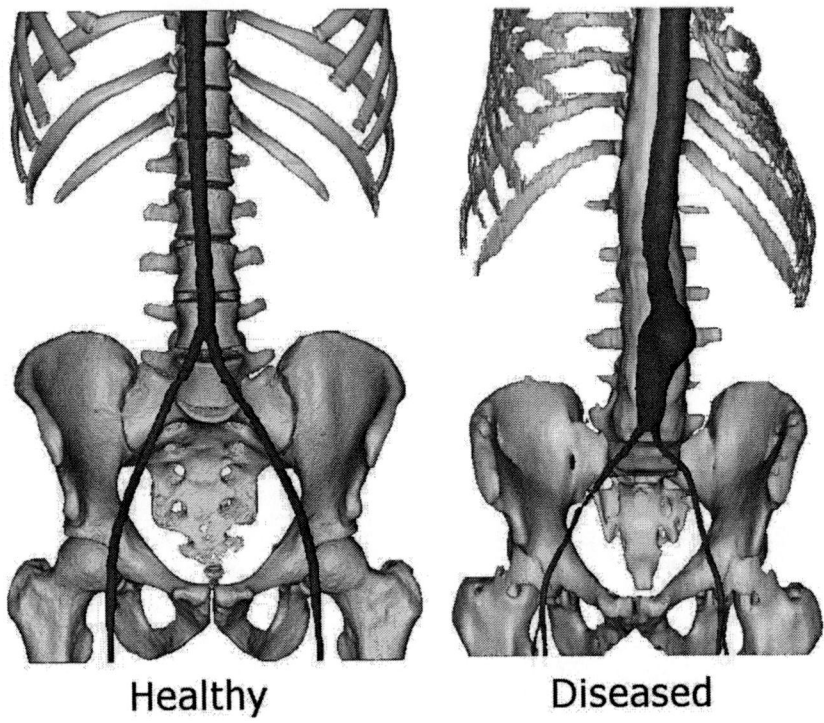

Figure 1. 3D reconstruction of a healthy *(left)* 28 year old male compared to a 76 year old male with an abdominal aortic aneurysm *(right)*. The differences between the two cases are clear to see, with the diseased case showing dilation and skewing of the aorta. Notice also the differences in skeletal structure due to age between the two cases.

With recent advancements in medical imaging technology, the recorded incidence of AAA is on the increase. It has been reported that over the last 30 years, AAA diagnosis has tripled in the Western world and this is likely to increase over the coming years as the average population age is on the rise [Bosch et al., 2001]. There are approximately 150,000 - 200,000 new cases in the US and 500,000 patients worldwide diagnosed each year. It is estimated that 1 million people worldwide are currently living with an undiagnosed AAA and that 95% of these cases could be successfully treated if detected prior to rupture. Mortality figures are also high, with a 95% mortality rate. These statistics contribute to rank AAAs as the 13th leading cause of death in the US and the 10th leading cause of death in men over the age of 55. Annually there are approximately 15,000 - 20,000 deaths in the US from AAA, and 8,000 deaths in the United Kingdom. The numbers of cases and subsequent deaths for Ireland is similar to international figures [Brosnan et al., 2009]. 30 - 50% of patients with a ruptured AAA die before they ever reach a hospital and even with surgical repair a 50 - 70% mortality rate remains. The condition is also more common in men than women, however, the disease is more lethal in women.

AAAs are typically asymptomatic and are usually detected through medical imaging as a result of unrelated health problems or screening programs of the elderly. Screening involves the use of ultrasonography to detect AAA and the implementation of these programs is becoming increasingly common. From a theoretical screening model of a population of 100,000 it has been estimated that 1500 lives could be saved, at a cost of $78,000 per life [Quill et al., 1989; Ernst, 1993]. Measurements of AAA size determined using ultrasonography are accurate up to 6 mm [Ernst, 1993], and therefore this approach has become the most cost-effective method of AAA detection. It has been recommended that people over the age of 60 - 65 years old, in particular men, should be screened for AAA, with the recommended age reducing to 50 - 55 when there is a history of aneurysmal disease in the family as this may increase the likelihood of AAA by up 6 times. AAA screening programs are becoming more widespread in the UK with many private institutions providing screening. The UK National Health Service (NHS) recently announced that a full screening program will be made available throughout the UK, but is unlikely to become widely available until 2013 [National Health Service, 2009]. Recently, it was suggested that AAA screening may be beneficial in Irish males aged 65 - 75 years [Brosnan et al., 2009]. According to the US Preventative Services Task Force [USPSTF, 2005], the potential benefit of screening for AAA among women over the age of 65 is low because of the number of age-related deaths in this population. The majority of AAA related deaths occur in women over the age of 80, and as there are many competing health risks at this age, any benefit of screening would be minimal [USPSTF, 2005]. Various lifestyle considerations can also affect the prevalence of AAA, such as smoking, diet and obesity; with people who fall into these categories may be more likely to either have or develop an AAA.

Upon detection of an AAA, there is currently much debate as how to best assess the severity and rupture risk of the patient. Currently, the trend in determining the severity of an AAA is to use the maximum diameter criteria [Cronenwett et al., 1985; Glimaker et al., 1991]. Patients with an AAA that has a maximum diameter greater than 5 - 5.5 cm are deemed a high rupture risk and are usually recommended for surgical repair [Lederle et al., 2002]. In the case of smaller AAAs where the diameter is <5 cm, the preferred approach is often careful and frequent observation using either ultrasonography or computed tomography (CT) scanning. Recent research however, has cast doubt over the suitability of surgical repair based on a maximum diameter criteria alone [Raghavan et al., 2000; Sayers et al., 2002; Fillinger et al., 2002, 2003; Vande Geest et al., 2006a; Kleinstreuer and Li, 2006; Leung et al., 2006; Doyle et al., 2009a, 2009b]. Although the diameter-criterion can be justified, as the rupture risk for an AAA is clearly related to its maximum diameter [Conway et al., 2001; Fillinger et al., 2002], surgical decision-making using the diameter-criterion alone may in fact lead to both unnecessary AAA repairs and also exclude certain cases (AAA <5 cm) from surgical repair [Darling et al., 1977; Cronenwett et al., 1985; Nicholls et al., 1998; Fillinger et al., 2002]. Nicholls et al. [1998] reported that 10 - 24% of ruptured AAAs were less than 5cm in diameter. Darling et al. [1977] also reported that of 473 non-repaired AAAs examined from autopsy reports, there were 118 cases of rupture, 13% of which were less than 5 cm in diameter. They also showed that 60% of the AAAs greater than 5 cm (including 54% of those AAAs between 7.1 and 10 cm) never experienced rupture. Vorp et al. [2008] later deduced from the findings of Darling et al. [1977] that if the maximum diameter criterion were followed for the 473 subjects, only 7% (34/473) of cases would have succumbed to rupture prior to surgical intervention as the diameter was less than 5 cm, with 25% (116/473) of cases possibly undergoing unnecessary surgery since these AAAs may never have ruptured.

Alternative methods of rupture assessment have been recently reported. The majority of these approaches involve the numerical analysis of AAAs using the common engineering technique of the finite element method (FEM) to determine the wall stress distributions. Recent reports have shown that these stress distributions have been shown to correlate to the overall geometry of the AAA rather than solely to the maximum diameter [Vorp et al., 1998; Sacks et al., 1999; Doyle et al., 2009a]. It is also known that wall stress alone does not govern failure as an AAA will rupture when the local wall stress exceeds the local wall strength. Therefore, rupture assessment is most suitable when both the patient-specific wall stress is coupled with patient-specific wall strength. A non-invasive method of determining patient-dependent wall strength was recently reported by Vande Geest et al. [2006b], with more traditional approaches to strength determination via tensile testing performed by others [Raghavan et al., 1996, 2006; Thubrikar et al., 2001a]. Newly proposed AAA assessment methods include: AAA wall stress [Fillinger et al., 2002, 2003; Venkatasubramaniam et al., 2004]; AAA expansion rate [Hirose et al., 1998];

degree of asymmetry [Doyle et al., 2009a]; presence of intraluminal thrombus (ILT)[1] [Wang et al., 2002]; a rupture potential index (RPI) [Vorp et al. 2005; Vande Geest et al., 2006a]; a finite element analysis rupture index (FEARI) [Doyle et al., 2009b]; biomechanical factors coupled with computer analysis [Kleinstreuer and Li, 2006]; growth of ILT [Stenbaek et al., 2006]; geometrical parameters of the AAA [Giannoglu et al., 2006]; and also a method of determining AAA growth and rupture based on mathematical models [Watton et al., 2004; Volokh and Vorp, 2008]. Based on these hypotheses, it is believed that an improved predictor of AAA rupture is desirable and may have clinical importance [Vorp et al., 1998; Raghavan et al., 2000a, 2000b; Sayers et al., 2002; Wang et al., 2002; Fillinger et al., 2002, 2003; Vande Geest et al., 2006b; Kleinstreuer and Li, 2006; Leung et al., 2006; Doyle et al., 2009a, 2009b].

Detection of AAAs by medical imaging leads to the clinical question: should the AAA be surgically repaired or monitored? Monitoring of AAAs, particularly smaller aneurysms, has been shown in the past to be effective, with the usual recommendations being repeat ultrasound every six months for AAAs 4 – 5 cm in diameter and every three months for larger AAAs [Ernst, 1998]. During this monitoring phase, expansion rates are also observed. If the expansion rate exceeds 0.5 cm per year, surgical intervention is often recommended. Further to aneurysm size deciding the fate of the AAA, other contraindications to elective repair are also commonly considered. These include, but are not limited to: myocardial infarction within the past six months; intractable congestive heart failure; intractable angina pectoris; severe chronic renal insufficiency, incapacitating effects from stroke, and a life expectancy of less than two years.

If the clinical outcome is to surgically repair the AAA, two approaches may be considered, both utilising a graft to exclude blood flow and pressure from the aneurysmal sac and return it to a relatively normal state. These options are either the traditional approach of open surgical repair or the minimally-invasive technique of endovascular aneurysm repair (EVAR). The gold standard in AAA repair is the open surgical method. The long-term durability of the procedure is excellent, with little need for post-operative intervention [Garcia-Madrid et al., 2004; Goueffic et al., 2005; Corbett et al., 2008]. However, this procedure is highly invasive and poses serious risk of complications during the operation [Sakalihasan et al., 2005; Vogel et al.,

---

1 Intraluminal thrombus (ILT) consists of a fibrin structure incorporated with blood cells, platelets, blood proteins and cellular debris, and are found in most AAAs.

2005; Corbett et al., 2008]. EVAR, on the other hand, is the preferred treatment in older patients and patients unfit for open repair. This procedure uses minimally-invasive techniques, entering the aorta via the femoral artery, resulting in minimal scarring, reduced blood-loss and a significant reduction in operation time. Questions have, however, been raised recently about the effectiveness of EVAR compared to open repair, in particular with regards to the biomechanical performance of the stent-graft resulting in post-operative complications such as endoleak, graft migration, and fabric tears [EVAR Trial Participants, 2005a; EVAR Trial Participants, 2005b; Corbett et al., 2008].

1.2. MEDICAL IMAGING

The term "medical imaging" commonly refers to the techniques and processes used to create images of the human body for clinical purposes or medical science. These purposes are often to reveal, diagnose or examine disease, or to study the normal anatomy and physiology of the human body. Over the last number of decades, medical imaging has advanced from the earliest forms of x-rays which began at the beginning of the 1900's to the more recent developments of sophisticated ultrasound and magnetic resonance imaging. Each imaging technique has its own strengths and weaknesses, and the method of imaging is typically defined by the desired application. For example, traditional ultrasonography is employed to image the foetus in pregnant women, as this technique is powerful enough to reveal the desired information regarding the foetus and with no health risk. More complex imaging techniques are required for detailed examination structures such as the cerebral arteries. In this case, magnetic resonance imaging (MRI) may be used. This imaging process allows excellent soft tissue contrast enabling detailed images of the blood vessels within the Circle of Willis to be captured. For the purpose of this chapter, medical imaging will focus on computed tomography as this is the medical imaging technique commonly employed for imaging cardiovascular disease and the 3D reconstructions of AAAs. CT, or computed axial tomography (CAT), uses helical tomography to produce two dimensional images of the structures in a thin section of the body through the use of x-rays. The technique is a non-invasive imaging procedure that utilises non-ionizing radiation to create high-resolution 2D images of the anatomy and is capable of differentiating between a wide range of tissues. CT is the gold standard for diagnosing many abdominal diseases, such as renal stones, pancreatitis, appendicitis, diverticulitis, bowel obstruction and AAA. For an in-depth description of the underlying mathematics and theories involved with CT imaging, one can refer to Webb [1990]. A typical CT image of an AAA can be seen in Figure 2. The AAA is easily distinguishable in the image, and these 2D cross-sectional images provide valuable information to the clinician regarding size and shape of the aneurysm. One drawback of traditional CT 2D images is the difficulty in obtaining accurate wall thickness information. This problem is evident in Figure 2, as the pixel intensity, measured in Hounsfield units (HU), of the diseased AAA wall is too similar to the ILT to determine wall thickness. It is possible in certain cases to determine the wall thickness based on the thickness of the calcifications embedded in the wall, but in cases where there are negligible calcifications, the problem remains.

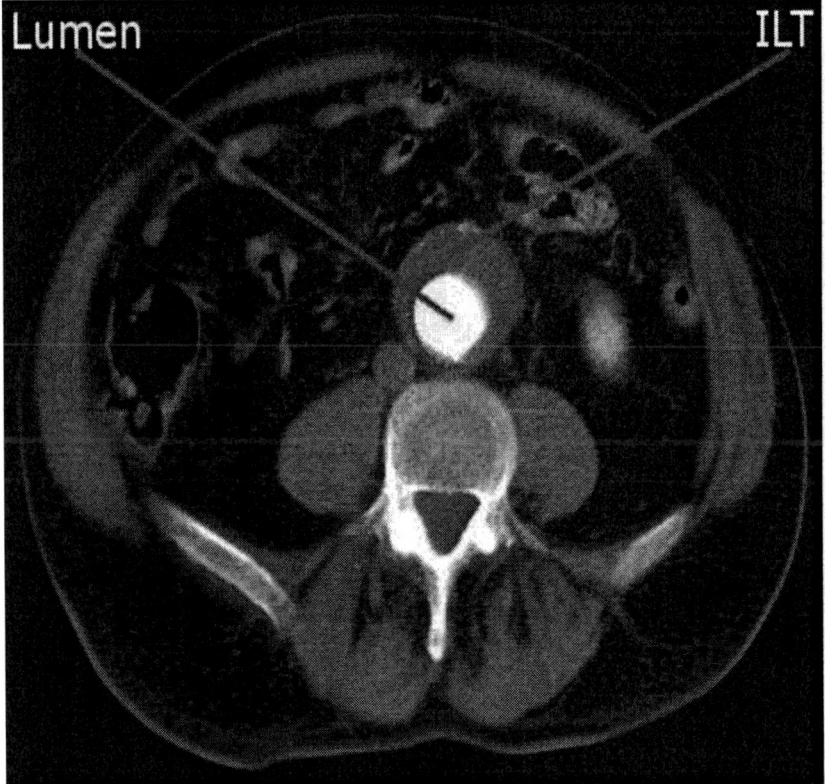

Figure 2. Typical CT scan of patient with AAA. AAAs predominantly form with ILT encapsulated between the lumen region and the diseased aortic wall.

Chapter 2

3D RECONSTRUCTION FROM CT SCANS

Further to 2D use of CT images, recent advancements in technology have enabled the reconstruction of 3D models from the 2D images. Numerous software programs are available nowadays from freeware to commercial programs, all of which are capable of essentially generating 3D reconstructions of medical images. The reconstruction software used throughout this chapter is the commercially available software Mimics v12 [Materialise, Belgium]. In order to actually reconstruct the 3D AAA from the 2D CT scans, many techniques are employed. Firstly, the CT scans in Digital Imaging and Communications in Medicine (DICOM) format are imported into the software. Once imported, the technique known as thresholding can be applied. The input to a thresholding operation is typically a greyscale or colour image, in this case greyscale CT scans. Thresholding is a useful method of separating out regions of an image that are of interest, from those that are background. This segmentation technique is often based on the different intensities or colours in the foreground and background regions of an image. When segmenting a CT scan, it is often useful to filter pixels whose intensity values lie within a certain range, or band of intensities. For this operation, black pixels correspond to background, and white pixels to foreground. Now, the image is segmented into regions of interest (white pixels) and background regions (black pixels). Instead of forcing foreground pixels to white, it is also possible to leave all pixels of interest as their original colour in order to preserve information.

As CT scans are complex images, they require more refinement than a simple thresholding operation. Whilst the thresholding is being performed, the software is employing an edge detection algorithm. Edge detection is a fundamental tool used in most image processing applications to obtain information from the frames as a precursor step to feature extraction and object segmentation. This process detects outlines of an object and boundaries between objects and the background in the image. The basic edge-detection operator is a matrix area gradient operation that determines the level of variance between different pixels. This edge-detection operator is calculated by forming a matrix centered on a pixel chosen as the center of the matrix area. If the value of this matrix area is above a given threshold, then the middle pixel is classified as an edge. There are many ways in which edge detection can be performed, with most being grouped into two categories; gradient and Laplacian.

The algorithm used in Mimics v12 is the *marching squares* and *marching cubes* algorithm. Marching cubes is one of the latest algorithms of surface reconstruction used for viewing 3D data, and was first described by Lorensen and Cline in 1987. This algorithm produces a triangle mesh by computing isosurfaces from discrete data. From connecting the patches from all the cubes on the isosurface boundary, a surface representation can be obtained. This high-resolution 3D surface construction algorithm produces models with unprecedented detail. These 3D reconstructions can be generated using a variety of algorithms, but the three more commonly employed techniques are shaded surface display, maximum intensity projection, and more recently, 3D volume rendering [Calhoun et al., 1999]. Mimics v12 utilises the 3D volume rendering approach, in particular, the OpenGL [Open Graphics Library, Silicon Graphics International] graphics language. This hardware acceleration offers high quality rendering including Gouraud shading for optimal display of the 3D objects. Gouraud shading is a method used in *computer graphics* to simulate the differing effects of light and colour across the surface of an object. The basic principle behind this OpenGL language is to define the volumetric data as a three-dimensional texture and render it by mapping it onto a stack of "display slices" that are orthogonal to the viewing direction [Tam et al., 1997; Cabral et al., 1994]. As a result of these algorithms within Mimics v12, detailed 3D reconstructions of medical images are possible. The use of additional techniques such as layering, allow reconstructions of exquisite detail to be produced. Figure 3 shows a typical reconstruction of anatomical structures from CT images, highlighting the use of layers to allow further use of the reconstructions by hiding/replacing certain regions of interest.

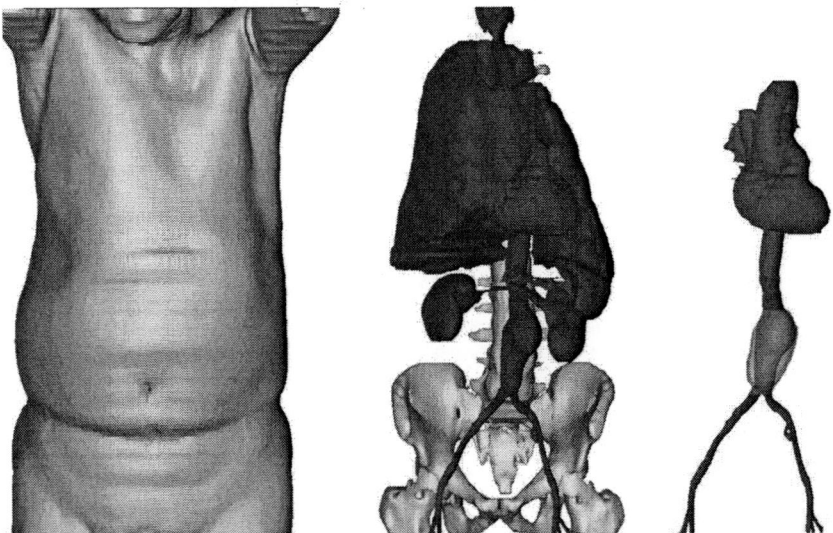

Figure 3. Full 3D reconstruction of CT scan data set. Image shows the use of layers to highlight/remove particular regions of interest such as organs and bones. Reproduced from Doyle et al. [2009c].

Chapter 3

APPLICATIONS OF AAA 3D RECONSTRUCTIONS

The resulting 3D reconstructions have many applications toward the further understanding of AAA disease. Over recent years these virtual AAA models have allowed researchers to apply numerical techniques such as finite elements analysis (FEA), computational fluid dynamics (CFD) and also fluid-structure interaction (FSI) to the problem, thus highlighting regions of complex stress distributions or irregularities in the haemodynamics. 3D reconstructions also allow experimental methods to be effectively employed, as reconstructions enable the creation of *in vitro* replications for bench-top testing. Whilst numerical techniques are the more commonly employed tools used by researchers for determining the severity of AAAs and the post-operative success of AAA stent-grafts, there remains a need for experimental methods in order to validate these numerical approaches. For the purposes of this chapter, the following work will branch into two distinct areas, that is, numerical and experimental investigations. Both avenues of research rely heavily on the 3D reconstruction method of the AAA and results can vary significantly depending on the technique used. Smoothing is essential on reconstructions to be used for further research so as to eliminate unwanted detail that will impair the quality of the results, but also ensuring that particular details are not lost due to over-smoothing. Overall, 3D reconstructions have advanced the treatment and therapy options available to patients in many areas of health and disease and now AAAs can benefit from similar advancements. The following sections of this chapter will identify and describe some of the more recent developments in the field of AAA biomechanics and 3D imaging form both a numerical and experimental viewpoint.

Chapter 4

NUMERICAL INVESTIGATIONS

The primary roles of numerical studies involving AAA include: 3D reconstructions of the AAA to determine the morphology and dimensions of the aneurysm for stent-graft sizing; evaluating the degree of asymmetry of the AAA and the resulting posterior wall stress; the determination of peak wall stress to assess the likelihood of rupture; examination of the fluid flow and resulting wall stress within the AAA both before and after surgical repair; the optimisation of stent-graft design in order to enhance stent-graft technology; analysis of the post-operative biomechanics of the stent-graft; and computer aided design (CAD) and computer aided manufacturing (CAM) to create experimental AAA models.

4.1. PRE-OPERATIVE PLANNING FOR EVAR

Pre-operative planning involves patient-specific 3D reconstructions of the AAA to determine the most suitable approach to EVAR. Upon reconstruction, the clinician can foresee any possible complications with the repair, in particular, problems with access sites and vessel geometry. As part of this chapter section, CT scan data was obtained from the Midwestern Regional Hospital, Limerick, and St. James's Hospital, Dublin, for 4 patients either awaiting or previously undergone surgical repair of an AAA. All patients were male with a mean age of 77.5 yrs (range 59 – 87 yrs). CT scans were obtained using a Somatom Plus 4 [Siemens AG, D-91052 Erlangen, Germany]. The mean pixel size of the CT scans was 0.675 mm with all scans taken using a 3 mm slice increment. The CT scans were imported into Mimics v12 for 3D reconstruction. For these particular reconstructions, only the lumen regions were of clinical importance as this is the region to which the stent-graft is deployed and fixated.

Reconstruction times can range from as little as 2 minutes for a basic model where minor details are ignored, to 1 hour where all details are included such as the ILT and surface indentations. The critical dimensions when concerned with EVAR stent-grafts are the neck diameter of the stent-graft, the iliac diameter, and also the length of the device. Clinician's can usually determine the neck diameter without difficulty using 2D CT scans, but problems can arise when determining length. 3D reconstruction allows the overall length to be easily measured, thus allowing the exact sizing of the medical device. The measurements are taken from below the lowest renal artery to a point in the iliac arteries where the clinician feels comfortable will maintain an adequate fixation of the device. A variety of measurements are possible from the reconstruction, as shown in Figure 4, with the clinician able to determine certain distances that can help overcome possible obstacles with the surgical repair. 3D reconstruction of one particular patient revealed an extremely tortuous proximal neck that may cause difficulties during the surgical procedure. 3D reconstruction highlighted the degree of curvature of the neck and allowed the clinician to decide on the most suitable approach before EVAR. As shown in Figure 4, the proximal neck of the AAA required special attention during the operation. As the upper portion of the stent-graft is embedded into the proximal neck, the tortuous nature of this could complicate placement and fixation of the device.

The patient-specific reconstruction shown in Figure 5 was a particularly extreme case. In this reconstruction, the full extent of the aneurysmal aorta was revealed. This patient had a descending thoracic abdominal aneurysm (TAA), abdominal aortic aneurysm (AAA) and also an iliac aortic aneurysm (IAA). For the case shown in Figure 5, the clinician decided to only repair the TAA with a stent-graft. This decision was solely based on surgical experience as the AAA had also exceeded the threshold for repair (diameter > 5.5cm).

The reconstruction of the stent-graft after placement within the TAA of Figure 5 can be seen in Figure 6. The device now excludes the region of high stress predicted using numerical tools and thus aids to return the aorta to a lower stress state that is relatively safe from rupture.

Numerical Investigations 17

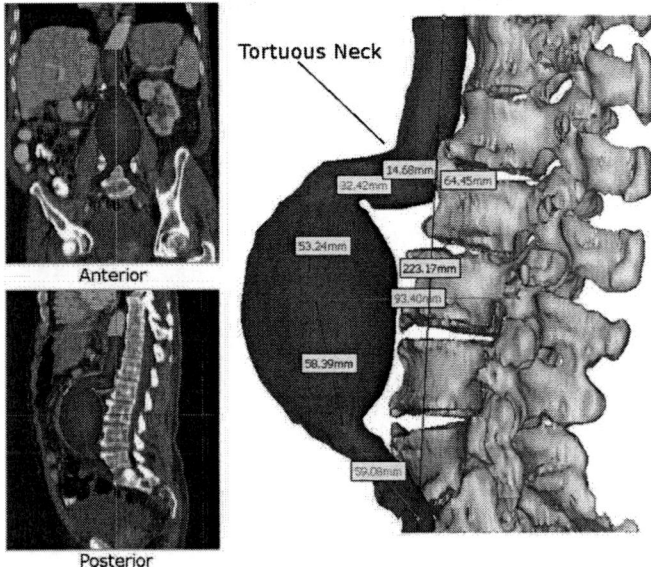

Figure 4. Example reconstruction showing measurements obtainable from reconstructions. All measurements are in millimetres (mm). The 3D reconstruction showed exactly the degree of tortuosity, allowing the clinician to decide on the most suitable means of approach during EVAR.

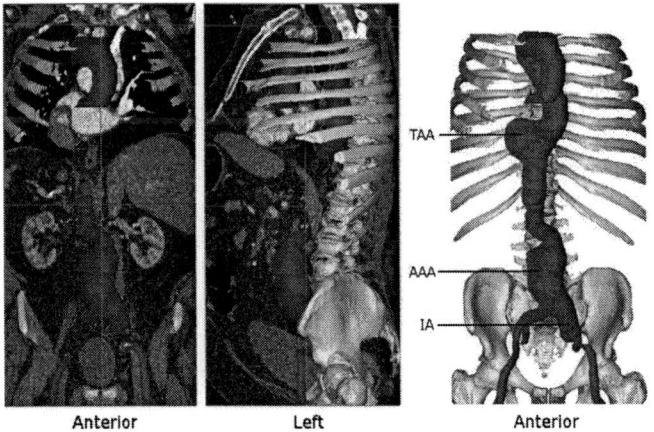

Figure 5. 3D reconstruction showing thoracic aortic aneurysm (TAA), abdominal aortic aneurysm (AAA) and iliac aneurysm (IA) from the anterior viewpoint. The patient had significant tortuosity of the aorta and aneurysms at three separate locations. The clinician decided to repair the TAA and monitor the growth of the AAA and IA.

This reconstruction was generated from post-operative CT scans that help to monitor the diseased aorta, and help highlight any additional aneurysm growth from endotension [EVAR Trial Participants, 2004], or further progression of the AAA. Post-operative 3D reconstructions can also aid the clinician to observe the outcome of the EVAR procedure at regular intervals. Stent-graft limbs can often become kinked, twisted or occluded by thrombosis [Corbett et al., 2008], which can complicate the flow of blood and may require further intervention by the clinician. Although these complications can be identified using 2D CT scans, 3D reconstructions allow exact visualisation of the problem and aid towards a better understanding of the overall situation of the patient. Currently, there is no institution-wide standard regarding stent-graft sizing, with many clinicians opting for their own methods of measurements, particularly lengths. There is still a degree of learning among the EVAR community when concerned with AAA morphology and stent-graft behaviour. The latest generation of the Medtronic Endurant™ graft appears to shorten more in length on deployment than its predecessor, Talent™, due to design modifications. This consequently affects the recommended measurements and sizing by the manufacturer. Ultimately, better imaging and 3D reconstructions can only add to the quality of the endovascular repair. The procedure is quick to perform and could not only help towards standardising the measurement and sizing of stent-grafts, but could also aid surgeons in improving the treatment of AAAs.

4.2. STENT-GRAFT DESIGN

Further to pre-operative planning of stent-graft sizing, 3D reconstructions also greatly aid with stent-graft design. As EVAR is becoming the favoured choice for repair procedures among clinicians, much research is aimed at identifying the limitations of both EVAR and stent-grafts [Parodi et al., 1991; Egelhoff et al., 1999; Kamineni et al., 2004; Corbett et al., 2008]. The primary complications with EVAR are graft migration, endoleaks and to a lesser extent thrombotic occlusion. It has been suggested that re-designing current stent-graft devices may provide a remedy to these problems. The design of conventional grafts and stent-grafts has normally featured a constant proximal diameter with a sudden diameter reduction at the bifurcation. In the healthy aorta this is not the case as the geometry tapers smoothly into the iliac arteries [Shipkowitz et al., 1998]. The rapid cross-section area change with conventional bifurcated devices causes the flow to converge, promoting flow separation and recirculation in the iliac limbs that may be associated with graft limb thrombosis [Chong and How, 2004; Jacobowitz et al., 1999]. Occlusions are believed to be caused by thrombosis as well as kinks, even though this is not a very common problem [Corbett et al., 2008].

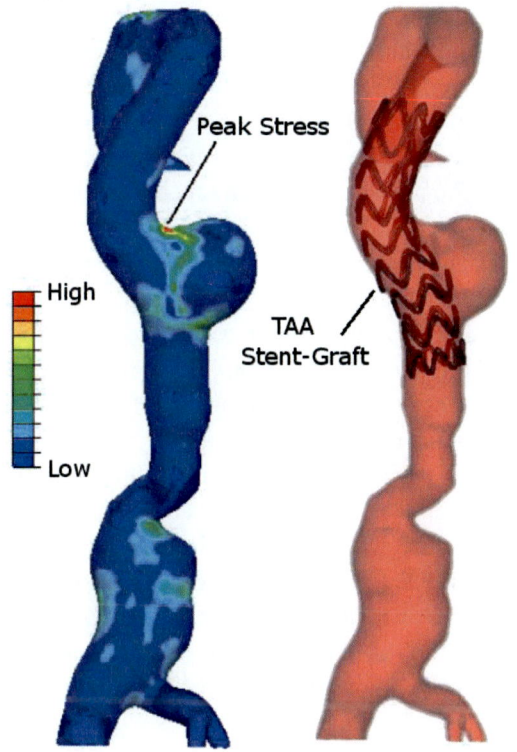

Figure 6. Illustration showing the pre-operative numerically predicted von Mises wall stress distribution *(left)*. Post-operative EVAR deployed TAA stent-graft *(right)* now excludes the TAA sac, returns blood flow in the descending aorta to a relatively normal state and reduces stress acting on the TAA wall. In this case, the clinician decided not to repair the AAA even though diameter > 5.5cm. Pre-operative wall stress somewhat validates this decision as the TAA was under significantly higher wall stress than the AAA. Transparency of the aorta in the image on the right allows easy visualisation of the medical device. Models are shown from the posterior viewpoint.

CFD is a numerical tool capable of modelling the haemodynamics of the arterial system. The procedure involves taking a geometrical description of the volume the fluid occupies and dividing it into a finite number of volumes. The governing equations for fluid mechanics are then solved for each volume to give a representation of the fluid flow and fluid forces acting within the volume. CFD has been used to examine stent-graft performance in the past, providing useful information on flow patterns and forces affecting the device [Li and Kleinstreuer, 2005a; Howell et al., 2007]. Drag forces, which act on stent-grafts as a result of shear and pressure forces over the pulse cycle, have been implicated in graft migration. Drag is dominated by arterial pressure and is influenced by several factors, such as iliac angle, neck angle, and neck diameter [Howell et al., 2007]. CFD can be a cost-effective method for investigating alternative stent-graft designs. Our group previously investigated the potential benefits of a newly designed tapered stent-graft that maintains an area ratio at its inlet equal to that at the bifurcation of the device [Morris et al., 2006]. This novel stent-graft design is shown compared to a conventional design in Figure 7. In an *in vitro* study, the tapered design was associated with a reduction in blood pressure compared to a conventional graft [O'Brien et al., 2008]. Further to this line of research, this novel tapered stent-graft was compared to a conventional bifurcated stent-graft using both ideal uniplanar and realistic out-of-plane model configurations.

The conventional stent-graft, whose dimensions were based on previous work [Morris et al., 2004a], has a sudden change in area at the bifurcation point (an area ratio of 2:1 with respect to the inlet and bifurcation), while the tapered stent-graft is characterized by a tapering section from the proximal neck into the iliac limbs. The novelty of this tapered design lies in the blended transition outward as the iliac limbs separate from the trunk, which achieves a 1:1 area ratio at the bifurcation point, i.e., the same area at the entrance of the stent-graft and at the bifurcation. In order to solve the fluid equations using CFD, the fluid was assumed as laminar, incompressible, and Newtonian [Di Martino et al., 2001; Morris et al., 2004a], which is an acceptable assumption for large diameter arteries. Blood was modelled with a density of 1050 kg/m^3 and viscosity of 0.0035 Pa·s [Scotti et al., 2007]. The graft walls were considered rigid, with no slip [Morris et al., 2006]. Velocity and pressure pulses at the inlet and outlets, respectively, resembled those recorded from a typical abdominal aorta over a cardiac cycle by previous authors who had assumed laminar flow for the velocity profile [Di Martino et al., 2001; Morris et al., 2004]. By comparing the results of the conventional and tapered stent-grafts, it was apparent that the tapered design alleviated some of the problems associated with the conventional design. The new design reduced velocities by 18% and 31% above and below the iliac bifurcation, respectively. A comparison of the velocity profiles and secondary flow profiles between the two stent-graft designs are shown in Figure 8. For the full comparative study between the effectiveness of the new tapered design over the conventional stent-graft, including the application within patient-specific cases, the reader can refer to Molony et al. [2008].

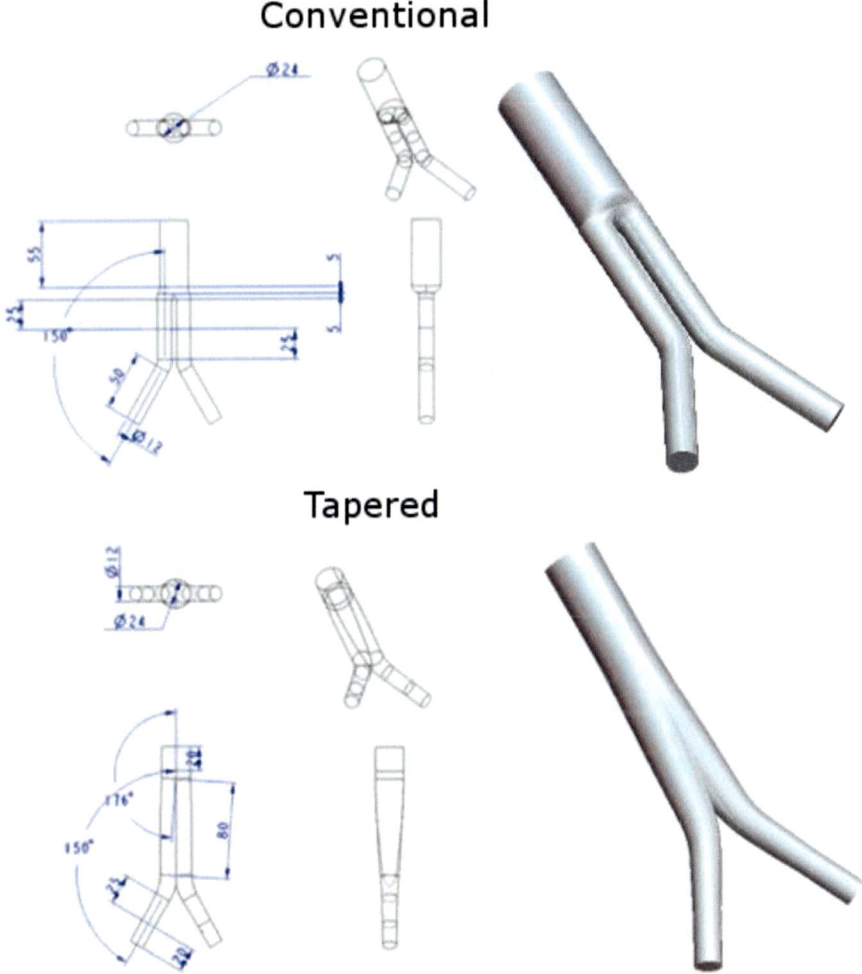

Figure 7. The conventional stent-graft design *(top)* compared to the novel tapered design *(bottom)*. The tapered stent-graft design maintains the area of the inlet throughout the bifurcation region, whereas, the conventional design has a rapid 2:1 area change at the bifurcation. This new smooth transition in area ratios has been shown to result in smoother velocity profiles and reduce secondary flows. Modified with permission from Molony et al. [2008].

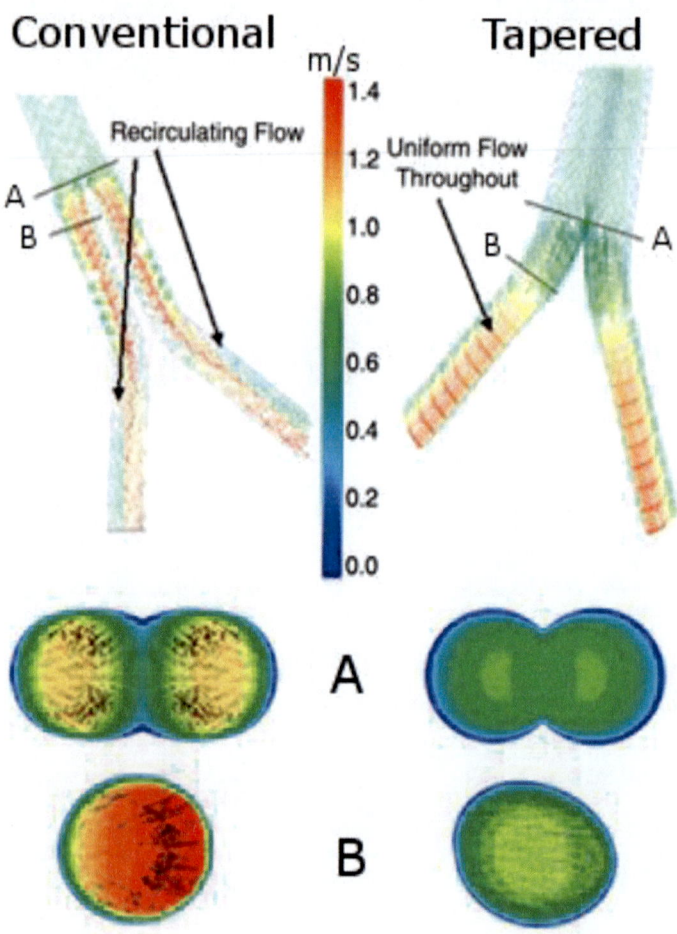

Figure 8. The axial velocity vector profiles (m/s) and cross sections showing secondary flows for the idealised models of the conventional and tapered stent-grafts. Modified with permission from Molony et al. [2008].

Based on CFD analysis, the novel tapered stent-graft improved graft haemodynamics compared to the conventional design. The tapered stent-graft reduced velocity and wall shear stress impinging on the graft wall and also resulting drag force. In the realistic scenario, the out-of-plane curvature reduces the positive impacts of the tapered design and thus, in patients with more irregular geometry, some of the benefits from the tapered design may be diminished.

4.3. OPTIMUM SMOOTHING OF 3D MODELS

Smoothing can significantly influence the resulting stress distributions in 3D numerical models. In order to determine the optimum level of smoothing applicable for these AAA models, an axial smoothing study was performed. The CT images were thresholded and segmented within Mimics, with polylines created at the boundaries of the segmentation. These polylines were then exported in IGES file format for further processing. Four full AAA 3D reconstructions of the same case were created and exported from Mimics. Each model was created using a different smoothing level by controlling the number of control points per axial polyline. FEA was then used to determine the wall stress on each model, helping to determine the optimum smoothing level. Artificial stress contours, and unrealistically high stress regions all indicate problems with the surface of the model. As shown in Figure 9, the wall stress contours of the four models revealed that at 20 control points per polyline is the optimum level of smoothing. Smoothing levels above 20 control points may unnecessarily smooth the surface removing important local details. Whereas, under-smoothing the models with control point number in excess of 20 may result in artificially high stressed areas and incorrect stress distributions. For a full description of the effect of modelling techniques on resulting AAA wall stress the reader can refer to Doyle et al. [2007].

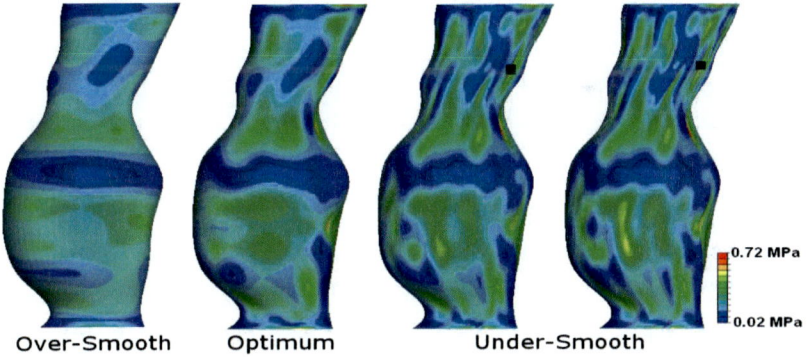

Figure 9: Axial smoothing study to determine the optimum number of control points per axial polyline. This test revealed that 20 control points per polyline is the desired level, as increasing this number over-smoothes the model, whereas, decreasing the number creates models with artificial stress distributions. The black mark in the under-smooth models indicates regions of artificially high wall stress. Reproduced from Doyle et al. [2007].

4.4. Determining AAA Asymmetry

Previous work [Vorp et al., 1998; Scotti et al., 2005] has identified the importance of asymmetry in idealised AAA models, and also indicated the need to investigate this aspect in realistic models. In this section, we have examined the role of asymmetry and resulting wall stress in realistic patient-specific AAA cases. Spiral CT scan data was obtained for 15 patients, comprised of 10 males and 5 females. Mean age ± standard deviation of the case subjects was 73.2 ± 6.7 years. These patient scans were obtained from the Midwestern Regional Hospital, Limerick, Ireland, and the University of Pittsburgh Medical Centre, Pittsburgh, PA, USA. All 15 patients were awaiting AAA repair, as AAA diameters had reached or exceeded the current 5 cm threshold for repair. CT scans were acquired using both the Somatom Plus 4 [Siemens AG, D-91052 Erlangen, Germany] and LightSpeed Plus [GE Medical Systems, General Electric Company] range of imaging equipment. All scans were single CT slices with a standard width x height of 512 x 512 pixels. Mean pixel size of scans was 0.742 ± 0.072 mm. The bodily structures of each subject were made visible using the non-ionic contrast dye, Optiray® [Mallinckrodt Inc., Convidien, MO, USA]. This CT data was then reconstructed using Mimics. These reconstructions allowed the computation of stress distributions within the geometries using the commercially available finite element solver ABAQUS [Dassault Systemes, SIMULIA, Rhode Island, USA]. The numerical tool of FEA involves dividing the structure into a smaller number of sub-domains, called elements. Each element is then connected via nodes. This series of elements over the surface and throughout the wall of the structure is known as a mesh. Certain constraints and boundary conditions are then applied to the model, typically to represent the conditions *in vivo*. Once adequate boundary conditions are in place, the software mathematically calculates the displacement of each node. From these displacements, stresses and strains are computed at integration points within the mesh, resulting in a full quantitative assessment of the stresses and strains within that particular AAA. Nowadays, this numerical tool is widespread among researchers in the assessment of AAA wall stress [Mower et al., 1997; Vorp et al., 1998; Raghavan et al., 2000; Di Martino et al., 2001; Thubrikar et al., 2001b; Hua et al., 2001; Wang et al., 2002; Fillinger et al., 2002, 2003; Venkatasubramaniam et al., 2004; Giannoglu et al., 2006; Leung et al., 2006; Papaharilaou et al., 2007; Speelman et al., 2007; Scotti et al., 2005, 2007; Truijers et al., 2007; Doyle et al., 2007, 2009a, 2009b, 2009c, 2009d; Rissland et al., 2009].

As CT scanning is routinely performed on AAA patients scheduled for repair, collection of this information involved no extra participation by the study subjects. All reconstructions were developed from scan positions immediately distal to the lowest renal artery to immediately proximal to the iliac bifurcation. The ILT was neglected in this study as with previous approaches [Vorp et al., 1998; Raghavan and Vorp, 2000; Thubrikar et al., 2001b; Fillinger et al., 2002, 2003; Scotti et al., 2005]. The thickness of the aorta wall is not easily identifiable from CT scans, therefore the wall was assumed to be uniform throughout the model and set to 2mm [Venkatasubramaniam et al., 2004]. This limiting assumption is one of the main concerns among researchers, as the AAA wall is known to be non-uniform in thickness, ranging from 0.23 – 4.26 mm [Raghavan et al., 2006]. All AAAs underwent the same degree of smoothing as previously reported by this author [Doyle et al., 2007]. The iliac bifurcation was omitted from this study, as in previous stress analysis work as it has been shown to not significantly affect the wall stress results of the AAA [Fillinger et al., 2002].

The AAA material was assumed to be homogenous and isotropic with non-linear realistic material properties [Raghavan and Vorp, 2000] that have been implemented in many previous publications [Sacks et al., 1999; Raghavan et al., 2000; Wang et al., 2002; Fillinger et al., 2002, 2003; Leung et al., 2005; Doyle et al., 2007; Papaharilaou et al., 2007]. The aorta is also known to be nearly incompressible with a Poisson's ratio of 0.49. The blood pressure within the AAA acts on the AAA inner wall and therefore, pressure was applied to the inner surface of the computational AAA model. A static peak systolic pressure of 120 mmHg (16 kPa) was used. In order to simulate the tethering of the AAA to the aorta at the renal junction and iliac bifurcation, the AAA model was fully constrained in the proximal and distal regions.

Most AAAs are constrained from radial expansion in the posterior direction due to the spinal column, therefore, AAAs predominantly dilate in the anterior plane. All cases studied in this analysis were naturally asymmetric in the anterior-posterior direction. In order to examine the effect asymmetry has on wall stress, the centreline of each AAA was automatically found using the reconstruction software. The centreline, which begins just below the renal arteries and ends immediately before the iliac bifurcation, passes through the centroid of each polyline slice in the series. Asymmetry is defined, in this case, as the perpendicular distance from the proximal and distal points of the centreline to a defined point on the centreline. Figure 10 shows how these asymmetry measures are obtained. Starting with the 3D AAA model in Figure 10A, a centreline is automatically created through the polyline centroids of

Figure 10B, thus creating Figure 10C. Then these polylines are exported from Mimics to ProEngineer Wildfire 3.0 [PTC, Lebanon, NH, USA]. Next, using the software, the end points of the centreline are connected with a straight line (Figure 10D) and a perpendicular line is extended from this connecting line, to predetermined points along the centreline (Figure 10E). The asymmetry at a specified distance along the AAA model is regarded as this perpendicular distance, and is measured in millimetres (mm). This method of determining AAA asymmetry results in a plot similar to that of Figure 10F which shows the normalised diameter plotted along the normalised length of the AAA.

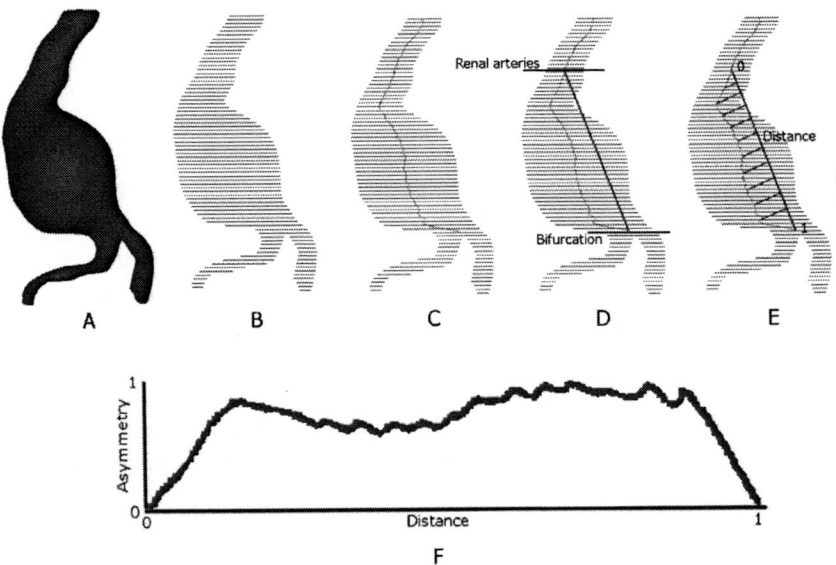

Figure 10. Illustration showing method used to obtain asymmetry measurements.

The results of this comparison revealed a strong relationship between the stress acting on the posterior wall and the degree of asymmetry in the anterior direction. In all cases studied, the relationship was evident, and as over 80% of AAAs rupture on the posterior wall [Darling et al., 1977], these findings may have clinical significance. For the full report of how posterior wall stress and asymmetry correlate, the reader may refer to Doyle et al. [2009a].

An alternative technique to measure asymmetry is also under development by the author. This tool uses the 2D CT images to directly determine asymmetry by simply comparing coordinates. The CT scan immediately below the lowest renal artery is examined, with the coordinates of the centre point of the AAA recorded. The clinician then follows through the series of CT scans until the scan revealing the most severe asymmetry is detected. This should be readily identifiable by experienced radiologists and clinicians. The coordinates of the centrepoint, or centroid, of the AAA at this region is again noted. Figure 11 shows the detection of centre points for the particular region of interest, that is, the AAA region of the CT scan. The 2D distance between these two points can then easily be determined by simply subtracting the Y-coordinates of each scan, resulting in a measurement of asymmetry in millimetres (mm). For the example shown in Figure 11, by subtracting the Y-coordinates, the resulting maximum asymmetry is approximately 25 mm. This allows the clinician to obtain a single parameter to assess the maximum degree of asymmetry of the particular AAA. The same method can be applied to each CT scan in the series if the full degree of asymmetry is desired along the length of the AAA, resulting in a plot similar to that shown in Figure 10F.

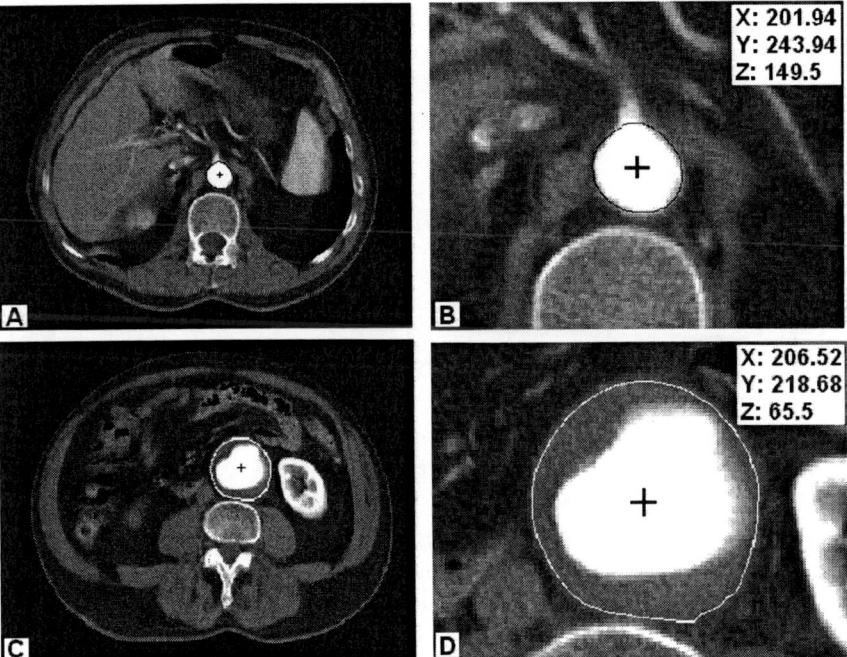

Figure 11. (A) CT scan depicting the proximal neck of the AAA with centre point identified, (B) Close-up view of region with centroid coordinates recorded, (C) Scan depicting the most severe region of asymmetry of the particular AAA, again with centroid shown, and (D) Close-up of scan with centre point coordinates recorded. Maximum asymmetry is 25 mm.

As mentioned previously, the majority of ruptures occur in the posterior region of the AAA. Based on these findings, both the diameter and asymmetry were statistically compared to posterior wall stress along the longitudinal distance of the aneurysm for 15 cases. This analysis was performed using a Spearman's Rho correlation bivariate test with significance defined as $P<0.05$. The results of this analysis are shown in Table 1.

Table 1. Correlation coefficients for posterior wall stress and both asymmetry and diameter

Patient	Asymmetry	P	Diameter	P
1	0.574	0.032	0.420	0.135
2	0.781	0.003	0.895	0.000
3	0.175	0.587	0.755	0.005
4	0.37	0.293	0.733	0.016
5	0.862	0.000	0.820	0.000
6	0.82	0.002	0.609	0.047
7	0.464	0.151	0.573	0.066
8	0.834	0.001	0.573	0.051
9	0.474	0.166	0.529	0.116
10	0.443	0.130	0.505	0.078
11	0.683	0.014	0.811	0.001
12	0.411	0.128	0.593	0.020
13	0.411	0.128	0.593	0.020
14	0.834	0.000	0.709	0.007
15	0.667	0.013	-0.132	0.668

The results are presented in Table 1 show how both asymmetry and diameter are comparable in their significance towards posterior wall stress. From the resulting correlations, 8/15 cases show asymmetry is significant and 9/15 cases show that diameter is significant. These results suggest that if posterior wall stress is to gain clinical acceptance as a possible high-risk rupture indicator, that both asymmetry and diameter may be as important in determining the posterior wall stress, and therefore may both equally contribute to AAA rupture. It has been previously postulated by Vorp et al. [2007] and also by Fillinger et al. [2002, 2003] that the biomechanics of the AAA may provide useful clinical guidance over the maximum diameter criteria. This present work supports this biomechanics-based approach and in particular suggests that posterior wall stress may be clinically important. The results presented also suggest that if peak wall stress is to remain the primary purpose of AAA stress analyses, then diameter remains a significant factor. It is also possible to apply this methodology to other potentially lethal aneurysms. Figure 12 illustrates how the asymmetry tool may be used to determine the asymmetrical nature of a TAA.

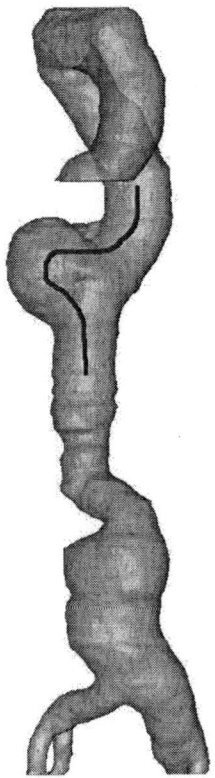

Figure 12. Image showing the centreline of a TAA which could be used to determine the level of asymmetry.

Although, ideally, stress analysis should be carried out on every AAA detected, the reality is that the decision to repair lies with the surgeon. The use of the maximum diameter criterion is very easy to implement for the surgeon, in that they must simply measure the maximum diameter from CT scans. The asymmetry condition described in this chapter could also be readily incorporated into the surgeon's decision making. This dilation, and ultimately asymmetry, can be identified by the clinician from basic 3D reconstruction, and could greatly aid in their decision to surgically intervene. Also, our group are developing an approach that accounts for asymmetry in all directions, and therefore the relationship between asymmetry and wall stress can be assessed in all AAAs, regardless of orientation. Once detected, the degree of bulging could be incorporated into the decision making process of the surgeon, and may refine and improve the current system of deciding on surgical intervention solely on the basis of maximum diameter.

4.5. IMPROVING RUPTURE PREDICTIONS

Currently, maximum diameter is the predominant factor governing AAA rupture risk, although, it is known that rupture will occur when the wall stress exceeds the wall strength. Therefore, the AAA tissue strength must play an equal role to AAA wall stress in determining failure. A region of AAA wall that is under elevated wall stress may also have high wall strength, thus equalising its rupture potential. The purpose of this section is to examine the use of a new additional tool to assist in the assessment of AAA rupture risk. This new approach focuses on a combination of the FEM coupled with published ultimate tensile strength (UTS) data from AAA tissue reported by previous researchers [Raghavan et al., 1996, 2006; Thubrikar et al., 2001]. This new approach, which we have described as the Finite Element Analysis Rupture Index (FEARI), may be clinically useful in aiding surgeons as to the most appropriate time to surgically intervene, and may serve as a useful adjunct to both maximum diameter and asymmetry.

As part of this study, CT scan data was obtained for 10 patients (male, n = 6; female, n = 4). These patient scans were obtained from the Midwestern Regional Hospital, Limerick, Ireland, and the University of Pittsburgh Medical Centre, Pittsburgh, PA, USA. All ten patients were awaiting AAA repair at the time of CT scan, as AAA diameters had reached or exceeded the current 5 cm threshold for repair. 3D reconstructions were performed, as previously described, using the commercial software Mimics. Patient-specific wall thickness was obtained using the equation proposed by Li and Kleinstreuer [2005b]. The ILT was also included in the reconstructions as this structure has been shown to reduce wall stress [Wang et al., 2002]. The models developed by this method formed the basis for the FEM stress analysis.

In order to simulate *in vivo* wall stress in the AAA wall, realistic boundary conditions were applied to each model. The AAA wall was modelled as a homogenous isotropic hyperelastic material using the finite strain constitutive model (Eqn.1) proposed by Raghavan and Vorp [2000].

$$W = C_1(I_B - 3) + C_2(I_B - 3)^2 \qquad \text{Eqn.1}$$

where, W is the strain energy density, I_B is the first invariant of the left Cauchy-Green deformation tensor and C_1 and C_2 are material coefficients based on population mean values ($C_1 = 0.174$ MPa and $C_3 = 1.881$ MPa). These material properties have been utilised in many previous stress analysis studies [Raghavan et al., 2000; Wang et al., 2002; Fillinger et al., 2002, 2003; Ventkatasubramaniam et al., 2004; Raghavan et al., 2005; Leung et al., 2005; Doyle et al., 2007, 2009a; Papaharilaou et al., 2007; Speelman et al., 2007]. The aorta is also known to be nearly incompressible with a Poisson's ratio of 0.49. The ILT was modelled as a hyperelastic material using the material characterisation derived from 50 ILT specimens from 14 patients performed by Wang et al. [2001] shown in Equation 2.

$$W = D_1(II_B - 3) + D_2(II_B - 3)^2 \qquad \text{Eqn.2}$$

where II_B is the second invariant of the left Cauchy-Green deformation tensor and D_1 and D_2 are population mean material constants derived for the ILT. Each AAA was constrained in the proximal and distal regions to simulate tethering to the aorta at the renal and iliac bifurcations. The blood pressure within the AAA acts on the luminal contour of the ILT and therefore, pressure was applied to the inner surface of the computational AAA model. A static peak systolic pressure of 120 mmHg (16 kPa) was used, as employed in most AAA stress analyses [Inzoli et al., 1993; Vorp et al., 1998; Giannoglu et al., 2006; Speelman et al., 2007; Truijers et al., 2007]. It is known that patient-specific blood pressures may be higher than 120 mmHg, but for the purpose of this study a standard value was more appropriate so as to eliminate some of the unknown variables in the analysis. Mesh independence was performed by increasing the number of elements in the mesh until the difference in peak stress was less than 2% of the previous mesh [Wang et al., 2002; Truijers et al., 2007; Doyle et al., 2007, 2009a]. This method of determining wall stress distributions has been previously shown to be the most effective in computing accurate results compared with other approaches [Doyle et al., 2007].

The FEARI is defined by Equation 3. In this equation, the peak wall stress is computed using the FEM, whereas, the wall strength values are obtained from previous research on experimental testing of AAA wall specimens [Raghavan et al., 1996, 2006; Thubrikar et al., 2001].

$$FEARI = \frac{\text{FEA Wall Stress}}{\text{Experimental Wall Strength}} \qquad \text{Eqn. 3}$$

This equation is based on the simple engineering definition of material failure and returns a value ranging from 0 to 1, where 0 indicates a very low rupture potential, and a value close to 1 indicates a very high rupture potential. In order to determine strength values for the AAA wall, the previous research of both Raghavan et al. [1996, 2006] and Thubrikar et al. [2001] were analysed. These publications are the most detailed reports of experimental uniaxial testing of AAA tissue. Raghavan et al. [1996] tensile tested 52 specimens of AAA tissue and found that the average UTS of this aneurysmal tissue was 0.942 MPa. Thubrikar et al. [2001] later segmented AAAs into posterior, anterior and lateral regions and tensile tested 49 tissue specimens. Average regional UTS values were shown to be 0.46 MPa, 0.45 MPa and 0.62 MPa, respectively. Raghavan et al. [2006] subsequently furthered their work, and also divided each AAA into regional sections and tested 48 samples. They showed that the UTS of AAA tissue can range from 0.336 – 2.35 MPa. They also reported that the regional variations in UTS for the anterior, posterior, left and right regions were 1.099 MPa, 1.272 MPa, 1.217 MPa and 1.224 MPa, respectively. By combining all the previously published experimental data, average regional UTS values for the four main regions of the AAA could be obtained. By subdividing the AAA into a further four sections, eight in total, more regionally accurate strength estimates were obtained, thus allowing FEARI values to be calculated. The method of dividing each AAA into regions is shown in Figure 13, with the resulting UTS values for the varying regions shown in Table 2.

Once the combined UTS values of AAA tissue were calculated, these values could be coupled with the computed wall stress results from the FEM. By recording the location of peak stress in each AAA model, the region can also be assigned a regional UTS value. FEARI was then computed for each of the ten cases. Statistical analysis was performed on all results using a Pearson's correlation test, with $P<0.05$ accepted as significant.

Table 2. Regional UTS values obtained by combining and averaging previous experimental data

AAA Region	UTS (MPa)
Anterior	0.7744
Posterior	0.8658
Left	0.9221
Right	0.9187
Anterior/Left	0.8482
Anterior/Right	0.8465
Posterior/Left	0.8939
Posterior/Right	0.8922

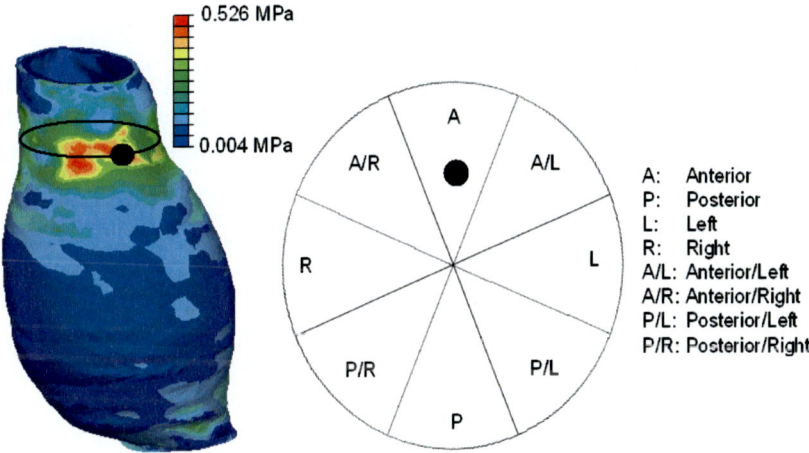

Figure 13: Illustration showing a representative AAA stress distribution for Patient 9 (ellipse passes through region of peak stress, indicated by black circle) and how each AAA model was segmented in order to determine the corresponding UTS value for the particular region of peak stress. In this case, peak stress occurs on the anterior wall of the AAA. AAA model shown in the anterior view. Reproduced from Doyle et al. [2009b].

By observing the stress distributions computed using FEA, it was noted that the regions of elevated and peak wall stresses occurred at inflection points on the AAA surface, and not at regions of maximum diameter. This observation was also observed by previous researchers in idealised models, both experimentally [Morris et al., 2004b; Doyle et al., 2009d] and numerically [Vorp et al., 1998; Callanan et al., 2004], and also in realistic models [Doyle et al., 2007, 2009a]. Inflection points are defined as points on the AAA surface at which the local AAA wall shape changes from concave outward to concave inward. The peak wall stresses found in this study ranged from 0.3167 – 1.282 MPa, with a mean ± standard deviation of 0.6201 ± 0.2836 MPa. The results of the computational stress analysis, along with the maximum diameter and UTS for each case can be seen in Table 3. There was no statistical significance between peak wall stress and any geometrical parameters analysed here. There was however a significant relationship between both FEARI and maximum diameter ($P=0.043$), and FEARI and AAA volume ($P=0.036$). The FEARI values observed using this new predictive tool for the ten cases examined are shown in Figure 14. This figure highlights the fact that AAAs with similar diameters may have markedly different rupture potentials, implying that maximum diameter is not a "one-size-fits-all" approach too AAA management.

Table 3. Maximum diameter, FEA computed peak wall stress, location of peak wall stress, and UTS of peak stress region in all ten cases examined. Wall thickness was incorporated in peak wall stress calculations

Patient	Max Diameter (cm)	Peak Wall Stress (MPa)	Location	UTS (MPa)
1	5.1	0.4291	Anterior	0.7744
2	5.8	0.3167	Left	0.9221
3	5.9	0.4346	Anterior/Right	0.8465
4	5.0	0.6641	Anterior/Right	0.8465
5	5.9	0.5866	Anterior/Right	0.8465
6	7.4	0.707	Right	0.9187
7	5.3	0.4	Anterior/Right	0.8465
8	6.2	1.282	Anterior	0.7744
9	6.5	0.5263	Anterior	0.7744
10	9.0	0.855	Posterior	0.8658

It is proposed that FEARI could serve as a useful adjunct to diameter-based surgical decision making. Diameter, and ultimately size of the AAA, is an obvious concern for the clinician and must remain a consideration. However, the overall geometry of the aneurysm should also play a role.

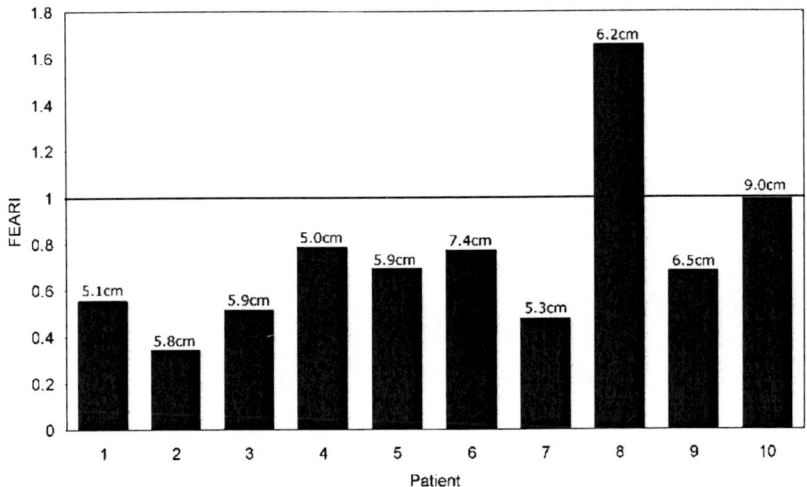

Figure 14. Graph displaying FEARI results for all ten cases. Horizontal line indicates possible AAA rupture based on the FEARI model. Diameters of each case are presented also indicating how diameter is not related to FEARI. Reproduced from Doyle et al. [2009b].

Asymmetry has been shown to affect wall stress in idealised AAA models [Vorp et al., 1998; Scotti et al., 2005] and may also affect realistic cases [Doyle et al., 2009a].

Other researchers have proposed the Rupture Potential Index (RPI) [Vande Geest et al., 2006a] which uses a statistical modelling technique with the inclusion of factors such as age, gender, family history, smoking status, among others, to deduce patient-specific wall strength [Vande Geest et al., 2006b]. This RPI approach uses a more theoretical method of calculating wall strength, compared to the experimental approach of FEARI, and combining the two approaches may lead to improved predictions. Ultimately, the decision to surgically intervene may include a combination of factors including diameter, asymmetry, RPI and FEARI, along with clinical experience, and may determine the most suitable approach to a particular AAA. FEARI may be clinically useful due to the simplicity of the approach. Rupture occurs when the AAA tissue cannot withstand the locally acting wall stress exerted, and therefore, tissue strength must be considered when assessing AAA rupture potential. Peak wall stresses were computed, along with the location, and therefore UTS, of peak wall stress region. FEARI results indicate that surgery may not be necessary for all cases, but rather continued monitoring may suit particular patients, although, at the time of this study all cases had received either traditional open repair or EVAR. It is proposed to couple FEARI together with diameter and other important factors in AAA assessment to allow the clinician a greater understanding of the severity of an individual AAA before deciding on surgical intervention. This preliminary study of a FEARI suggests that further work into this approach may yield more accurate results, and may provide a useful adjunct to the diameter-based approach in surgical decision-making.

4.5. PRE AND POST-OPERATIVE BIOMECHANICS

Within this section, the biomechanics in a pre- and post-operative patient-specific AAA are examined. The relatively new approach of FSI was employed to determine not only the wall stresses that contribute to rupture, but also the haemodynamics involved in both the diseased vessel and post-operative stent-graft. For this particular study, CT scan data for one AAA case was obtained from the HSE Midwestern Regional Hospital, Limerick, Ireland. The pre-operative scan is used to identify the aneurysm and ILT, whereas, the stent-graft can be identified in the post-operative scan. The space between ILT and the stent-graft is assumed to consist of stagnant blood. Cross sections were segmented from just below the infrarenal aorta to the beginning of the internal iliac arteries, similar to the previously described methodology. 3D reconstructions of these geometries were then exported to Gambit [ANSYS, Canonsburg, PA, USA] for mesh generation. Here both the fluid (lumen) and structure (aneurysm wall, thrombus and graft wall) domains are meshed, with the meshes then imported to Fluent 6.3.26 [ANSYS, Canonsburg, PA] where the solid region can then be exported to ABAQUS v6.7.

FSI is normally achieved either through a monolithic (full coupling) or partitioned approach (loose coupling) [Vierendeels et al., 2007]. The commercial software Mesh-based Parallel Code Coupling Interface (MpCCI) 3.0.6 [Fraunhofer SCAI, Germany] was used in this work. The software is based on the loose coupling of two chosen software's, namely, Fluent (fluid) and ABAQUS (structure). This approach allows the use of familiar and mature solvers for each domain. The benefits of using mature solvers are advanced capabilities that may not be available in monolithic solvers such as the use of non-linear material models, contact and interaction of surfaces and non-Newtonian fluid models.

For this application, data was exchanged every 0.005 seconds, with Fluent sending the pressure to ABAQUS, and ABAQUS sending the deformed nodal coordinates to Fluent. Fluent uses the Arbitrary Lagrangian Eulerian (ALE) method to deal with the deforming mesh. Specifically, a remeshing technique is used where cells are remeshed based on whether they violate a user specified size and skewness criteria. Both codes share a common boundary where the data exchange occurs. MpCCI identifies nodes or elements near each other based on an association scheme and data is then transferred from one node to the other. The software also allows for non-matching meshes, useful in complex applications such as the AAA. Further information is available to the reader in the MpCCI documentation [Fraunhofer SCAI, 2008].

The ILT and AAA wall were assumed to be hyperelastic, homogenous, incompressible and isotropic. The AAA wall and ILT were modelled using the constitutive models proposed by Raghavan and Vorp [2000] and Wang et al. [2001] and presented as Equations 1 and 2 in Section 4.5. It has been shown that the use of population mean values does not significantly affect the prediction of stresses on the aortic wall [Raghavan and Vorp, 2000]. The aneurysm and ILT were assigned values of 1120 kg/m^3 and 1121 kg/m^3 for the structural density respectively [Li and Kleinstreuer, 2005a]. The stent-graft was modelled as one whole body due to the difficulty in accurately reconstructing the nitinol stents from the CT data. Future advancements in 3D imaging may alleviate this problem. A Young's Modulus of 10 MPa and a density of 6000 kg/m^3 were assumed for the stent-graft [Li and Kleinstreuer, 2005a]. The graft and artery were assumed to be tied together, simulating attachment of the stent-graft to the artery wall, thus ignoring the possibility of endoleaks and local dislodgement.

The structural model consisted of 75,849 tetrahedral elements which were used both for the aneurysm and thrombus and 19,024 hexahedral elements used for the stent-graft. The space between the ILT and stent-graft was modelled with 21,974 hydrostatic pressure elements within ABAQUS. These simulated the stagnant blood in the aneurysm sac. The aneurysm inlet and outlets were constrained in all degrees-of-freedom. For the fluid boundary conditions, a velocity inlet was assigned while at the outlets a pressure boundary was assigned. The flow rate and blood pressure were not available for this particular patient and so previously published data was used [Mills et al., 1970]. Peak systolic flow occurred at 0.305 s and the peak systolic pressure occurred at 0.4 s. Blood was assumed to be a Newtonian fluid with a density of 1050 kg/m^3 and a viscosity of 0.0035 Pas [Scotti et al., 2007]. The PISO (Pressure Implicit with Splitting of Operators) algorithm was used for pressure-velocity coupling and the QUICK (Quadratic Upwind Differencing Scheme) scheme for discretisation of each control volume. The pre-operative lumen consisted of 231,000 tetrahedral elements, while the post-operative lumen (stent-graft) had 141,000 tetrahedral elements.

The pre-operative peak wall stress was found to be 0.38 MPa, which was reduced by 92% to 0.03 MPa in the post-operative case. Figure 15 illustrates the results of the FSI simulation. Peak wall stress occurred on the posterior wall both pre- and post-operatively. The pressure of the stagnant blood in the aneurysm sac varied from 0.001 MPa to 0.0015 MPa over the course of the cardiac pulse. The maximum stress in the aneurysm was observed in the neck region where the stent-graft is in contact with the aneurysm wall. The stress in the stent-graft is much greater than the stress in the aneurysm and this is shown by the grey values of Figure 15.

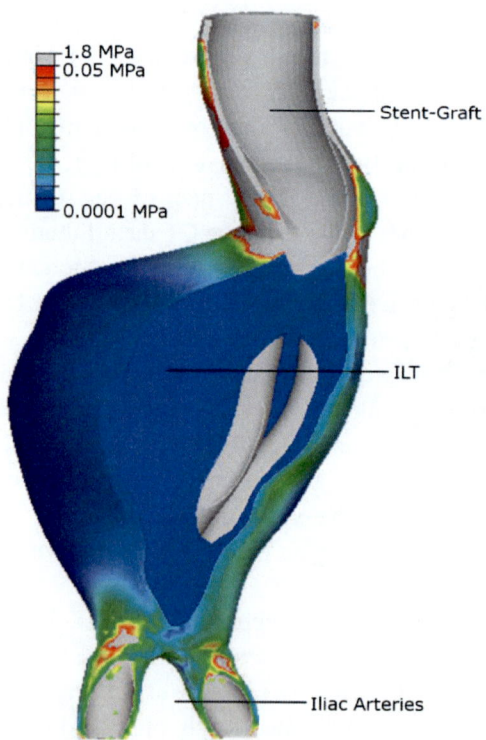

Figure 15. Cut-away view of the post-operative AAA model at t = 0.43 s of the cardiac pulse. This illustration shows how the stent-graft shields the aneurysm wall from higher stresses.

During peak systolic pressure the flow of blood has begun to decelerate, which can lead to vortex formation [Scotti et al., 2007]. The velocity pathlines and pressure contours around this time-point for the pre- and post-operative models are quite similar, as seen in Figure 16. One noticeable difference is the removal of a vortex after the graft has been implanted. This occurs just after the blood flow leaves the aneurysm neck (indicated by arrow in Figure 16). A greater pressure gradient can be seen in the post-operative model when compared to the pre-operative model. This correlates to approximately a 250 Pa greater pressure drop in the stent-graft. This large pressure gradient may be due to the curvature of the iliac limbs of the stent-graft. The drag force, which can lead to post-operative complications, is caused by pressure and viscous forces acting on the stent-graft [Morris et al., 2006a]. Peak drag force occurred prior to the peak systolic pressure with a value of 4.85 N and varied from a value of 2.85 N to 4.85 N over the cardiac cycle. Both the viscous force and pressure force followed the same trend as the velocity and pressure waveform respectively, with the majority of the force generated due to the pressure component. At peak systolic flow the viscous force was 1.1% of the total drag force, while at peak systolic pressure it was 0.35% of the total drag force.

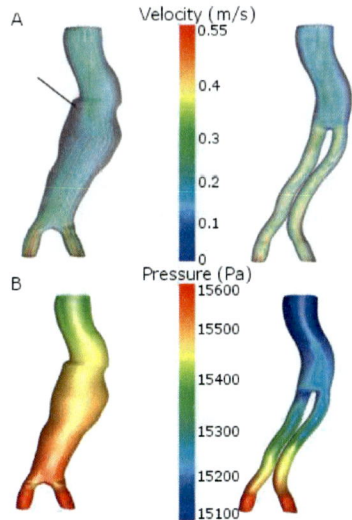

Figure 16: Velocity pathlines and pressure contours. (A) Velocity pathlines (m/s) for the pre-operative (left) and post-operative (right) cases, and (B) pressure contours (Pa) for the pre-operative (left) and post-operative (right) cases. These results are taken at the time of maximum wall stress (t = 0.4). The arrow indicates the presence of a vortex.

Fluid-structure interaction is a powerful tool available to researchers to identify both the wall stresses and haemodynamics within patient-specific AAAs. By combining both the structural and fluid elements of the AAA, the most accurate numerical predictions can be obtained. The work presented here on a pre and post-operative case study has revealed the effectiveness of EVAR as a surgical repair technique, and can also aid in highlighting any possible complications that may arise. The ability of FSI to compute the realistic drag forces acting on the stent-graft is of great benefit to clinician, as this information could help to evaluate the likelihood of graft migration which could lead to further problems such as sac re-pressurisation.

4.5. COMPUTER-AIDED DESIGN AND COMPUTER-AIDED MANUFACTURE

In order to compliment numerical tools and ultimately validate computationally derived results, experimental models are required. Advancements over recent years in computer technology allow 3D reconstructions from medical data sets to be further developed. CAD and CAM systems now enable virtual 3D models to become a reality. Although there are a number of CAD/CAM techniques available to researchers today, this section will describe a procedure for the methodology of converting 2D CT images into 3D CAD/CAM designs ready for machining. These machined moulds can then be used with the lost-wax injection-moulding process to produce anatomically-correct experimental models. Realistic experimental models can be used, not only in stress analyses such as the photoelastic method [Morris et al., 2004b], but also for fluid dynamics studies and post-operative experimental testing, such as stent graft distraction testing. The models are created by first reconstructing a virtual AAA model, leading to mould design, and then to manufacturing via the injection-moulding technique. Previous research has examined the use of rapid-prototyping as a method of producing elastomeric replicas of arterial vessels [Seong et al., 2005]. This method, although quick and effective, does not produce the surface finish that can be achieved using the injection-moulding process. Surface finish is of paramount importance when using arterial models for experimental testing using the photoelastic method, such as that previously conducted at our laboratory [Morris et al., 2004b]. Other techniques have been employed in order to make models for use in laser-Doppler anemometry

(LDA) [Loth et al., 1997] and PIV flow studies. This section describes the modelling and manufacturing processes used and to determine the effectiveness of the technique. This method of converting a standard CT scan to a patient-specific silicone model may be of value to many researchers in this field.

Polylines created in Mimics are imported into ProEngineer Wildfire 3.0. Surfaces are then recreated along these polylines. These surfaces are then split using its centreline into two exact halves, thus creating a two-piece mould set used in the manufacturing technique. Each patient-specific mould design consists of two sets of moulds. The first mould is designed to produce the casting wax model of the AAA, and the second set to produce the outer silicone model. The outer mould is approximately 2 mm larger in all regions than that of the wax mould, so as to produce a silicone model with a 2 mm thick wall. As the wall of an AAA can range in thickness from 0.23 – 4.33 mm [Raghavan et al., 2006], a wall thickness of 2 mm is a reasonable assumption and has been used in previous studies [O'Brien et al., 2005].

Each outer mould design includes supports for the inner wax cast to ensure location of the wax model inside the larger outer mould. Moulds can be designed that include or omit the iliac arteries. For experimental studies involving stress analyses, the iliac arteries are believed to be unimportant, whereas, for fluid dynamics and stent-graft testing, the iliac arteries are necessary to include. Moulds designed without the iliac arteries have cylindrical sections included both in the proximal and distal regions of the AAA, to allow attachment to experimental test rigs. Inclusion of the iliac arteries can significantly increase the complexity of the design as iliac arteries are often not on the same plane and so ensuring that the complete model is split into two exact halves with no gaps or overlaps is difficult to achieve.

Once the mould sets have been designed using CAD, the files are exported again in IGES format and imported into the software package AlphaCAM [Planit Holding Ltd., Kent, UK]. Within this software, the toolpath commands used to control the milling machine can be generated. Each mould is set-up with the same reference points so as that each mould piece fits together exactly, ensuring the resulting model has an almost negligible seamline. Machining is performed by a three-axis computer numerical control (CNC) milling machine using the machining codes generated within AlphaCAM. Moulds are machined from solid aluminium blocks (Figure 17) and are finished by hand to remove any unwanted burrs that results from the milling process. Necessary holes, guide pins, gates and vents can be added to each model during the machining procedure. For a detailed description on the CAD/CAM process see Doyle et al. [2008a].

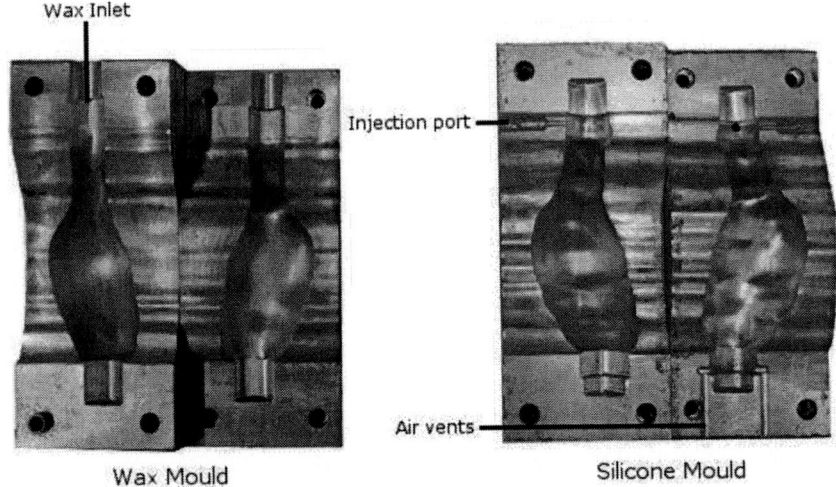

Figure 17. Example CNC-machined aluminium AAA moulds.

Chapter 5

EXPERIMENTAL INVESTIGATIONS

While CAD/CAM systems are used to design anatomically-correct virtual 3D models, manufacturing techniques allows these virtual models to become a reality. This section will describe a procedure for the methodology of manufacturing bench-top models of AAAs for use in various forms of experimental testing. This chapter describes models created using silicone rubber, yet this technology is applicable to any material that can be injected in a liquid state.

5.1. IN-VITRO MODELS

The procedure to actually make the experimental model is outlined as follows and detailed in full in Doyle et al. [2008a]. Over recent years the process has been refined to its current state through research into various manufacturing techniques. Initially, work began layering the silicone rubber onto an AAA phantom, a technique which has proved successful for some researchers in their efforts [Flora et al., 2002]. This method resulted in models with poor surface finish as shown in Figure 18. As surface finish is important for studies such as the photoelastic method and rupture testing, a more effective method was desired and achieved.

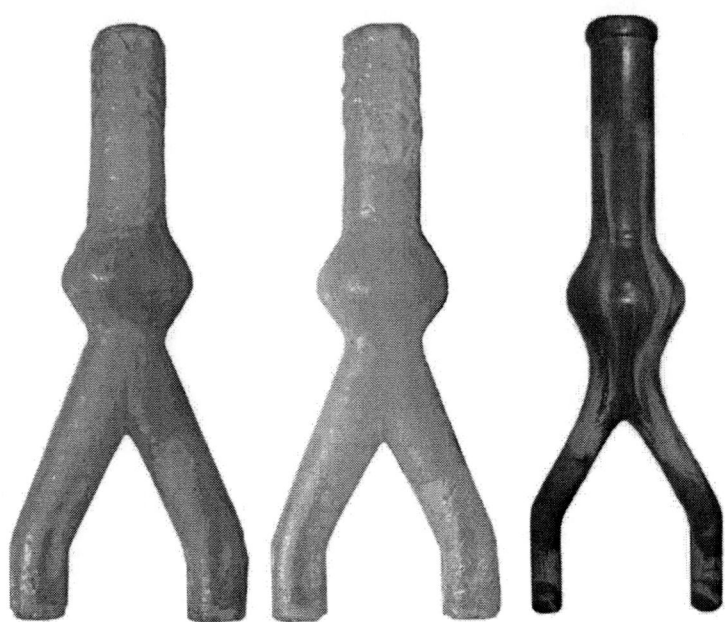

Figure 18. Evolution of the resulting silicone AAA models. Initially (*left and centre*) the material was layered onto a phantom resulting in a model with uneven and rough surface finish. Current techniques allow the creation of excellent AAA analogues (*right*), ideal for a variety of experimental studies. Notice the difference in iliac leg diameter near the bifurcation region due to the layering of the silicone.

All mould pieces were cleaned using acetone prior to use, with the wax moulds preheated to 40°C to minimise the contraction of the wax upon pouring. A casting wax, [Castylene B581, REMET Corporation] was used to make the lumen casts. The lumen casts were then placed into the outer moulds, which were coated with mould releasing agent [Ambersil Formula 8, Chemcraft Industries Ltd, Dublin, Ireland] and then clamped tightly together. The silicone rubber was then prepared, and slowly injected into the outer mould. The mould is then placed into an oven at a temperature of 50°C and cured for 24 hours. Once cured, the model is removed and the temperature is increased to 100°C in order to melt the wax from the mould. The resulting silicone model is then thoroughly cleaned, dried and inspected for defects.

Once manufactured, models should be examined for accuracy. As part of a quality check on the resulting silicone models, four models were assessed for wall thickness, one of which included the iliac arteries (Patient D). This study was performed by cutting each model longitudinally and measuring the wall thickness at distinct locations along the length of each model. The silicone models are designed to have a uniform 2 mm wall, but due to the contraction of the wax upon solidification and the expansion of silicone upon curing, a perfectly uniform wall is difficult to achieve. Tables 4 and 5 present the wall thickness results of this study and reveal that even though deviations in wall thickness do occur, the resulting percentage differences are within acceptable limits.

Table 4. Averaged wall thickness measurements at four locations on the AAA wall

		Axial Position			
		Anterior	*Posterior*	*Right*	*Left*
Patient A	Average Wall Thickness (mm)	1.87	1.97	2.09	2.55
	Standard Deviation	0.276	0.314	0.173	0.327
	Percentage Difference	6.95 %	1.78 %	4.23 %	21.47 %
Patient B	Average Wall Thickness (mm)	2.12	2.29	2.09	2.31
	Standard Deviation	0.207	0.418	0.235	0.248
	Percentage Difference	5.82 %	12.56 %	4.26 %	13.42 %
Patient C	Average Wall Thickness (mm)	2.18	2.17	2.53	2.30
	Standard Deviation	0.223	0.293	0.352	0.306
	Percentage Difference	8.08 %	7.89 %	20.99 %	13.09 %
Patient D	Average Wall Thickness (mm)	2.65	2.11	2.38	1.97
	Standard Deviation	0.653	0.282	0.414	0.281
	Percentage Difference	24.73 %	5.19 %	16.11%	1.64 %

Table 5. Averaged wall thickness measurements for each patient-specific AAA model

	Average Wall Thickness (mm)	Average Percentage Difference
Patient A	2.12	4.24 %
Patient B	2.20	9.01 %
Patient C	2.29	12.51 %
Patient D	2.22	11.09 %

These reproducible silicone models can be utilised for experimental testing of: vessel hemodynamics with LDA or PIV; wall stress analyses using either the photoelastic method or digital image correlation (DIC); and stent-graft studies by measuring dislodgement and drag forces, all of which may contribute to experimental validation of numerical work. In general, rubber models of good geometrical accuracy can be produced by sensible mould design and the use of controlled parameters in the silicone production. Models showed a maximum percentage difference of 9.21% between the designed moulds and the resulting silicone models. Overall, 3D reconstruction and CAD/CAM techniques proved to be successful in the replication of patient-specific rubber AAA models, and may help contribute to the use of patient-specific AAA models in experimental testing.

5.2. THE PHOTOELASTIC METHOD

Following on from the previous report from our group [Morris et al., 2004b] describing the use of the photoelastic method to determine the stress and strain in the idealised AAA model, this section will briefly examine the tool when applied to realistic AAA geometries. The experimental models were manufactured as outlined Section 5.1 and Doyle et al. [2008a] using PL-3 liquid photoelastic material and PC-11 reflective coating (Vishay Measurements Group UK Ltd., Hants, UK). For a full description of the methodology involved with the photoelastic method the reader can refer to Morris et al. [2004b]. In this study a static air pressure was applied to the internal surface of each model instead of the pulsatile cardiac loading previously used. Figure 19 compares the isochromatic fringes on the anterior wall of a patient-specific AAA under increasing loading conditions. The figure shows the fringe contours increasing as the pressure loading increases. Each fringe colour can be related to a fringe number (N) using a calibration chart, with N determining the relative stress and strain at a particular point. In Figure 19, the legend refers to the fringe number. Low fringe numbers will correspond to low stress/strain quantities. Figure 19 also reveals the complex contour distributions observed using the photoelastic method. Complex stress distributions have been witnessed in numerical stress analyses of AAAs and the use of the photoelastic method could serve as a useful technique to not only validate computational studies, but also provide researchers with an additional tool to determine the wall stress and strain of a patient-specific AAA.

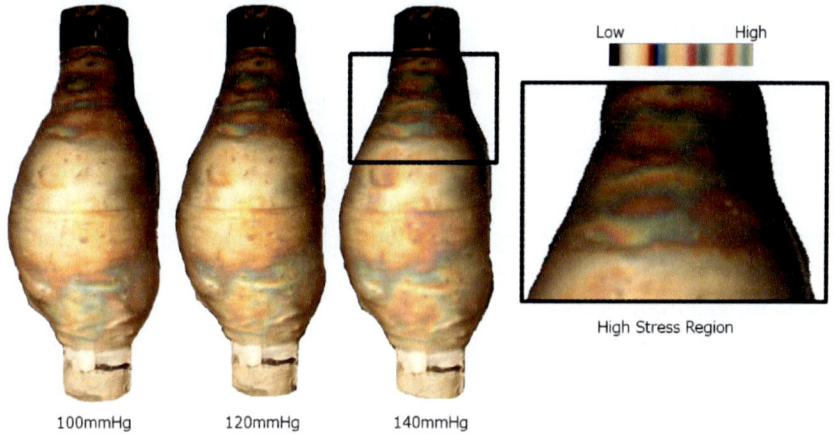

Figure 19. Isochromatic fringes on the anterior surface of a realistic AAA geometry.

5.3. IMPROVING EXPERIMENTAL MATERIALS

With the current technology in place to produce repeatable patient-specific AAA experimental models, it is desirable to improve the material analogues used to create these models. Currently, bench-top models are predominantly created using a homogenous material, often silicone, to represent the vessel wall. The diseased wall of the AAA in vivo is known to have a varying range of material strengths, with reports of the range in UTS to be from 0.34 – 2.35 MPa [Raghavan et al., 2006]. As AAAs can are non-homogenous in UTS, AAA analogues should also be ideally non-homogenous in strength. This section describes an effective method of creating a range of novel silicone rubbers that are linked to material strength through the colour of the material. This relationship is via calibration curves which effectively predict the strength of the silicone rubber when compared to the actual measured strength of the material.

5.3.1. Material Selection, Development and Testing

The commercially available Sylgard silicone from Dow Corning was chosen as the base material for this study, in particular, Sylgard 160 and Sylgard 170. These silicones were identified as appropriate materials as each material is easily identifiable due to its colour, and importantly, they have dissimilar material properties. Sylgard 160 is naturally grey in appearance with UTS of 4 MPa, whereas, Sylgard 170 is naturally black in colour with a UTS value of 2 MPa. These two materials were mixed together in various ratios in order to create a range of new silicones, with gradually increasing colour intensity from grey to black and gradually decreasing failure properties from 4 – 2 MPa. The ratios of each mix were increased by 10% for each new silicone, resulting in 11 complete materials, including the original Sylgard 160 and 170.

The colour intensity of each silicone was analysed using a ColorLite sph850 Spectrophotometer [ColorLite GmbH], allowing each silicone mix to be assigned an individual colour intensity value (ΔE). Colour measurements are given in as a variation of ΔE (Eqn. 4), where pure black has a ΔE value of zero.

$$\Delta E = \left[\Delta L^2 + \Delta a^2 + \Delta b^2 \right]^{\frac{1}{2}} \qquad \text{Eqn. 4}$$

Uniaxial tensile testing was performed using a Tinius Olsen H25KS [Tinius Olsen, Ltd., Surrey RH1 5DZ, England] with a 1 kN load cell. Each material was formed into Type 2 dumb-bell specimens conforming to BS ISO 37. Each sample was subjected to a cross-head speed of 500 mm/min [BS ISO 37], with a preconditioning of 10 cycles to 20% of the gauge length. Preconditioning helps to increase repeatability of the tests by stabilising the stress-strain function of the material. The structural properties of elastomers change significantly during the first several times that the material experiences straining. This behaviour is commonly referred to as the Mullins effect [Mullins, 1969]. The primary purpose of the tensile testing in this application was to generate force-extension data, which can be converted to stress-strain data, and determine the UTS of each silicone mixture.

Tear testing was performed using a modification of the trouser test pieces outlined in BS ISO 34-1. The Tinius Olsen was again used for this analysis. A cross-head speed of 100 mm/min was applied to each sample as per BS ISO 34-1. Tear testing results in tear strength (TS) values, which provide an indication of the resistance of the material to tearing, with results given in force per unit length. On failure of the specimen, the tear resistance, or tear strength, is calculated by Equation 5.

$$TS = \frac{F}{t}$$ Eqn. 5

where: TS is the tear strength (N/mm); F is the maximum load (N); and t is the specimen thickness (mm). By relating the colour intensity of each material to its respective UTS and TS, calibration curves could be generated. These curves then allow the UTS and TS to be predicted for that particular material based on the colour intensity. These curves are shown in Figures 20 and 21 with the values tabulated in Table 6. Significant correlations between results were assessed using a non-parametric Spearman's Rho bivariate correlation test using SPSS 15.0. Correlation coefficient (CC) is shown where significant relationships were observed.

Table 6. Results of the colour analysis, tensile testing and tear testing. All results are averages of the sample size

	Tensile Testing		Tear Testing	
Silicone Type	ΔE	UTS (MPa)	ΔE	TS (N/mm)
160	47.72	3.822	45.73	0.697
10:90	40.16	3.537	40.74	0.68
20:80	36.91	3.599	37.23	0.754
30:70	31.92	3.289	34.52	0.692
40:60	32.52	2.611	31.32	0.688
50:50	29.88	3.206	28.54	0.573
60:40	27.33	2.473	28.76	0.537
70:30	26.41	2.445	26.39	0.479
80:20	25.13	2.199	25.40	0.519
90:10	24.55	2.401	23.79	0.433
170	23.86	2.077	23.84	0.452

Good linear relationships were shown between both ΔE and UTS (R^2=0.8082), and ΔE and TS (R^2=0.7205). It was also possible to examine how accurate these calibration curves are in predicting the material property. This was achieved by manufacturing identical batches of silicone rubber at each concentration. The colour intensity of each sample was then measured, and together with the calibration curves, could be linked to a particular strength.

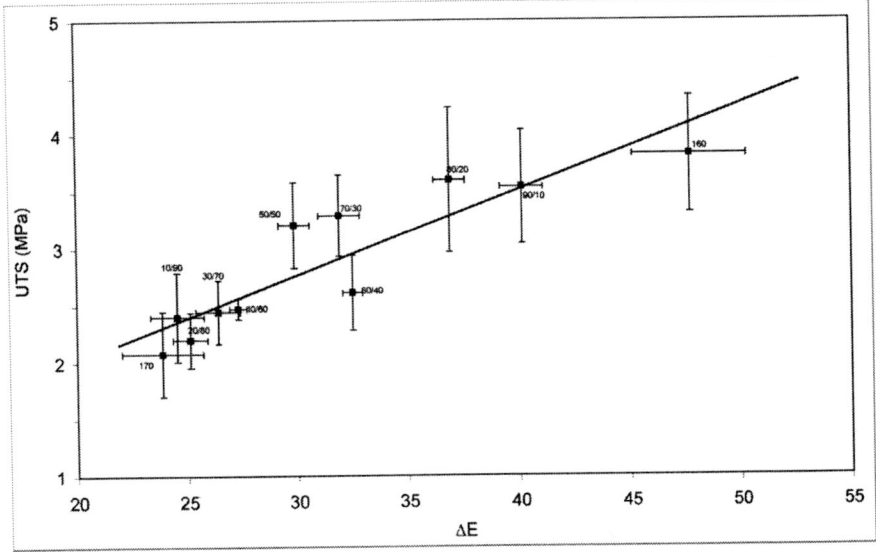

Figure 20. UTS calibration curve showing the new relationship between ultimate tensile strength and the colour of the material. Each data point is named with the corresponding material type. Reproduced from Doyle et al. [2009e].

In order to mechanically characterise each material so that they could be incorporated into numerical software, the experimental force-extension data from the tensile tests were converted to engineering stress and engineering strain. A 2nd order polynomial curve was applied to the data to obtain a mean experimental data curve. This mean data was then applied to the commercial FEA solver ABAQUS v.6.7 in order to find the most applicable strain energy function (SEF), and allow the determination of material coefficients. Material coefficients were then assessed using a Type 2 dumb-bell numerical model. The model was examined using identical boundary conditions to those applied experimentally. The stress and strain at a central node was then mapped throughout the course of the analysis, and compared to the results found experimentally.

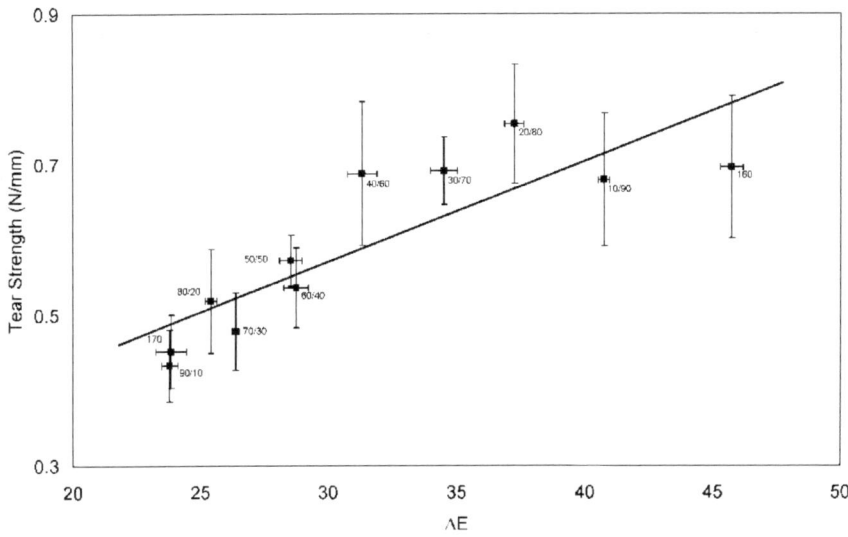

Figure 21. TS calibration curve showing the how tear strength relates to the colour of the particular material. Each data point is named with the corresponding material type. Reproduced from Doyle et al. [2009e].

The comparison between experimentally derived results and the numerical results obtained with the new material coefficients for the novel silicone rubbers is shown in Figure 22. Good linear agreement was observed between the predicted values and the measured values for both the UTS (R^2=0.8882) and the TS (R^2=0.8089). Overall, the predicted UTS and measured UTS results were significant (CC=0.945, p<0.0009), as were the predicted TS and measured TS results (CC=0.891, p<0.0009). The UTS results and tear strength results were also compared which showed a good linear trend (R^2=0.7318) and significant relationship (CC=0.9, p<0.0009) between the two material properties. This allows tear strength to be related to UTS for each varying silicone material thus giving a further insight into the relationship between the two properties. For a full description of the characterisation, SEF coefficients and development of these materials the reader can refer to Doyle et al. [2009e].

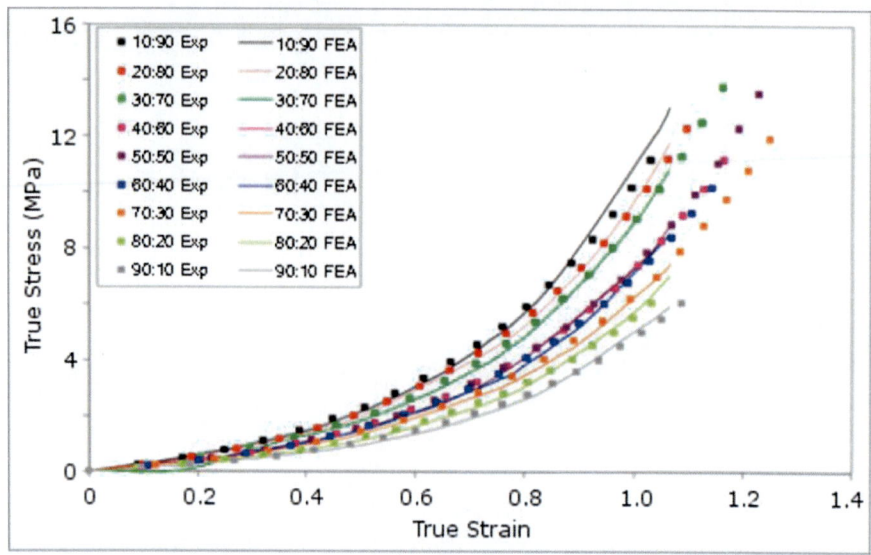

Figure 22. True stress and true strain for each of the nine novel materials developed from Sylgard 160 and Sylgard 170. Good agreement was observed between the experimental tensile result and the numerical results using the new SEF material coefficients.

5.3.2. Application to 3D Geometries

Idealised AAA silicone models were manufactured using a previously reported technique [O'Brien et al., 2005; Doyle et al., 2008a]. These analogues were designed to have realistic dimensions based on population averages obtained from the EUROSTAR data registry [Laheij et al., 2001] where the maximum outer diameter is 54 mm. This ideal AAA model has been utilised in previous research by our group [Morris et al., 2004b; Callanan et al., 2004; O'Brien et al., 2005; Doyle et al., 2008b, 2009d, 2009e]. Three models were created using Sylgard 160, three using Sylgard 170, and one model was created by randomly injecting both Sylgard 160 and Sylgard 170 through a Y-tubing connection into the wall cavity. This allowed both silicones to randomly mix via the injection process, resulting in a model of random material properties and various shades of black and grey. Examples of these models can be seen in Figure 23.

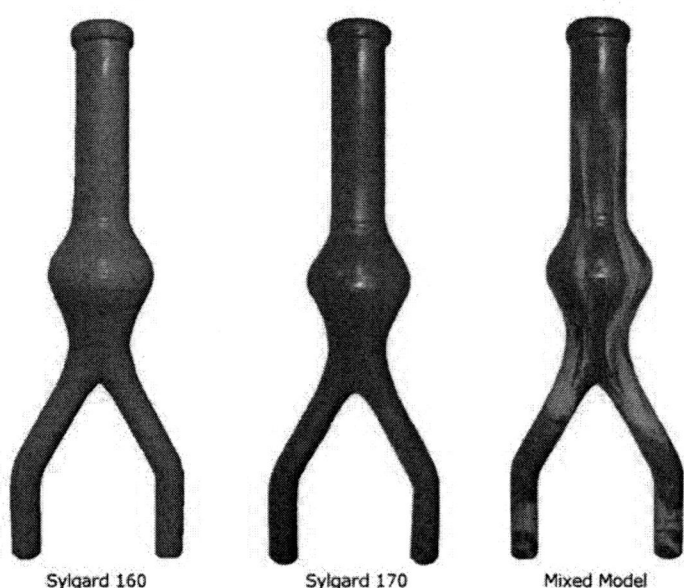

Figure 23. Example images of ideal AAAs made using Sylgard 160 (grey), Sylgard 170 (black) and a mixture of the two materials. Reproduced from Doyle et al. [2009e].

These experimental models were then used in conjunction with the non-contact strain measurement technique of videoextensometry to measure the change in diameter of each model under certain loading conditions. Each model was loaded with an internal pressure increasing from 0 mmHg to 160 mmHg in 20 mmHg increments. The models were constrained from movement at the proximal neck and iliac legs representing the attachment to the aorta *in vivo*. The diametrical change of each model was recorded with the results then averaged. These measurements were performed with the Messphysik Materials Testing Videoextensometer 1362CA [Messphysik Materials Testing, Austria] in conjunction with the Messphysik Dot Measurement for Windows software. The initial maximum diameter of each model was 54 mm, and so any displacement past 54 mm at each pressure loading is recorded with the software.

The ColorLite sph850 Spectrophotometer was used to measure the colour intensity of the mixed ideal AAA model with measurements taken at 20mm intervals along the length of the model, at the front, back, left, and right sides. These measurement locations are shown in Figure 24. The results show how the ΔE value differs depending on the concentration of either Sylgard 170 or Sylgard 160.

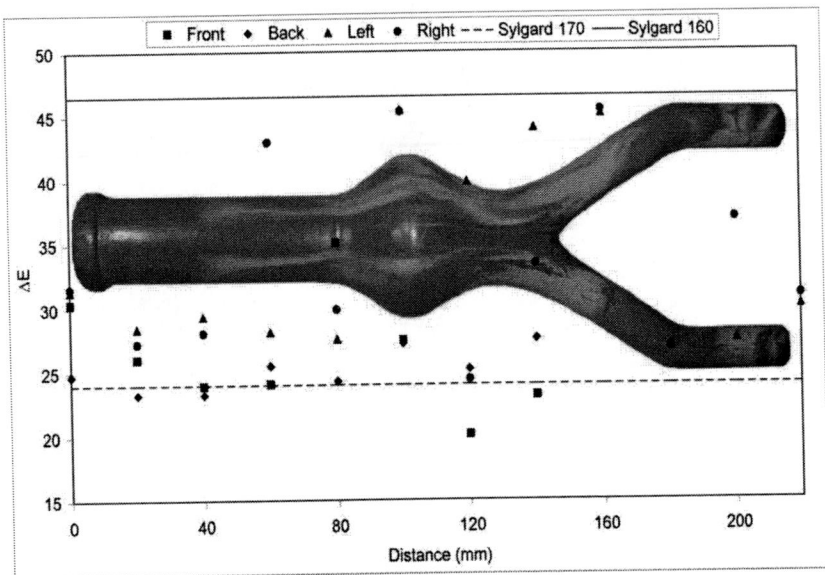

Figure 24. Colour intensity measurements along the four sides of the mixed ideal AAA model. The figure shows the random distribution of ΔE values dispersed throughout the model. Mean ΔE values for pure Sylgard 160 and Sylgard 170 are shown for comparison.

In order to assess the effectiveness of the material coefficients derived as part of this study and their applicability to 3D geometries, the videoextensometry experiment was replicated using the finite element method. The numerical model has a uniform wall of 2 mm, and was constrained from movement at the proximal neck and iliac legs, reproducing the experimental set-up. A half model was examined due to the symmetrical nature of the idealised AAA. The model was meshed using 11,443 quadratic tetrahedral 3D stress elements, with mesh independence achieved by increasing the mesh size until the peak stress was <2% of the previous mesh [Wang et al., 2001; Doyle et al., 2007; Truijers et al., 2007]. The same loading conditions were applied to the inner surface of the model and the displacement of the maximum diameter region was measured at each loading. By measuring the displacement at the region of maximum diameter, the deformation of the experimental models could be compared to those observed numerically. The experimental and numerical results were statistically highly significant for the Sylgard 160 model (CC=1.0, $p<0.0009$), Sylgard 170 model (CC=1.0, $p<0.0009$) and also the mixed silicone model (CC=0.971, $p<0.0009$). Overall, there was a difference in the diameter change of 0.24% (range 0.01 - 1.78%) and 0.38%

(range 0.3 - 5.27%) for the Sylgard 160 and Sylgard 170, respectively. For the mixed ideal AAA model, deformations were only measured from the front of the model, as with the experimental model, with an average percentage difference of 0.76% (range 0.25-5.03%). The results can be seen in Figure 25.

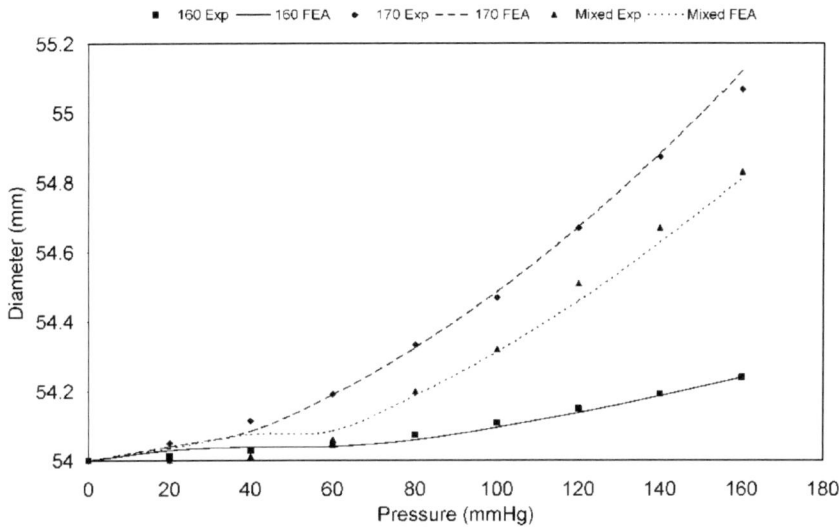

Figure 25. Experimental and numerical results for the pressure-diameter tests on the idealised AAA model. Good correlation between the two methods was observed for each model type. Reproduced from Doyle et al. [2009e].

Based on Section 5.3.1 and 5.3.2, it is now possible to create experimental AAA models with a variation of wall strengths throughout the model. Each wall strength can be effectively linked to a certain material model, which can be accurately modelled numerically.

5.4. EXPERIMENTAL RUPTURE TESTING

Following on from the developments described in Section 5.3, experimental models and novel silicone rubbers can be employed in experimental rupture tests. In recent publications by Doyle et al. [2008b and 2009d], which are the first known reports on experimental AAA rupture, a methodology used to accurately capture the location of rupture was described. These articles described a technique using high-speed photography to determine exactly where an experimental model will rupture, with accurate numerical predictions computed using FEA. In these previous studies, it was shown that idealised AAA geometries rupture at inflection points on the surface of the model, with these inflection points defined as areas where there curvature changes from concave to convex. The comparison between experimental rupture and numerically predicted peak wall stress can be seen in Figure 26.

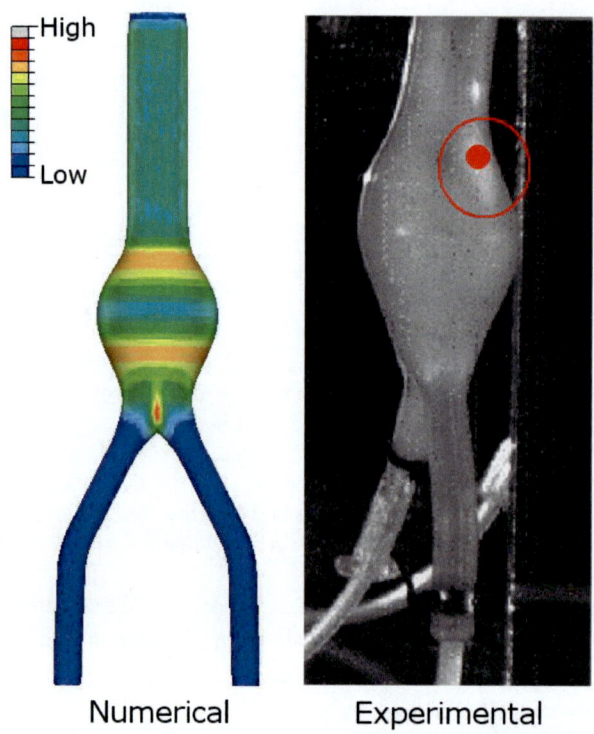

Figure 26. Numerical results compared to the experimental rupture test. Shown are the von Mises stress contours on the deformed idealised model compared to a snapshot of the moment of rupture. The numerical results shown high stresses at the inflection regions with the experimental model rupturing at the proximal inflection point (marked in red). Modified from Doyle et al. [2009d].

Following on from the work described thus far led to the experimental rupture technique being applied to several realistic AAA geometries using the materials developed in Section 5.3. This entailed creating 16 patient-specific AAA silicone models based on the 4 geometries shown in Figure 27. These models consisted of 8 Sylgard 160 (grey) models and 8 Sylgard 170 (black) models. A further 5 models were also created (see Figure 28) using the mixing technique described in Section 5.2.2 to produce models with randomly distributed materials with properties that can be determined using spectrophotometry.

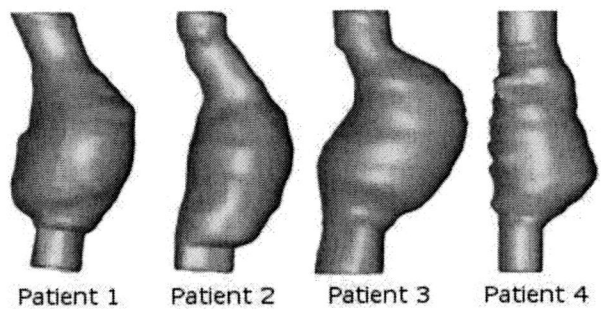

Figure 27. Realistic AAA geometries of the four patients used in the study.

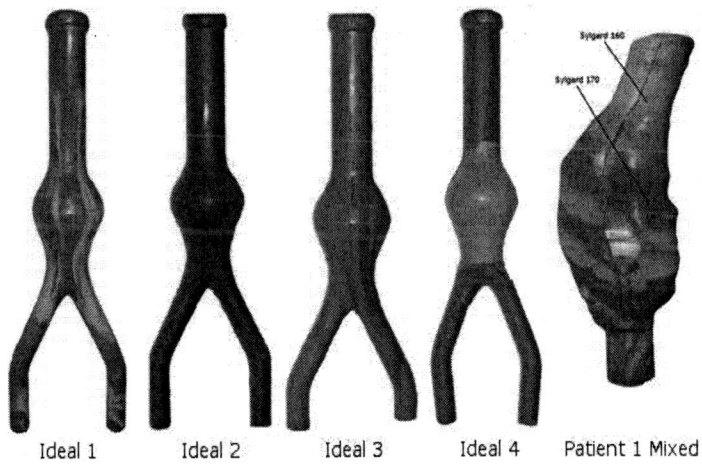

Figure 28: Illustration of the models created using the mixing technique described in Section 5.3.2. Ideal 1 is a random distribution, Ideal 2 is predominantly black, Ideal 3 is predominantly grey and Ideal 4 is a banded model with the AAA sac made using the stronger Sylgard 160 material. Patient 1 Mixed is a realistic AAA with randomly distributed materials.

An experimental test rig was adapted from literature [Doyle et al., 2008b, 2009d] allowing each model to be connected to a pneumatic air source and inflated to the point of rupture. A high-speed camera [Photron Fastcam SA1-1, Photron USA Inc.] was used at a frame rate of 2,000 frames per second (fps) enabling the point of rupture to be accurately captured. This particular camera is capable of recording at frame rates up to 675,000 fps. The positioning of a series of mirrors surrounding the experimental model allowed a full 360° view of the model, ensuring that the position of rupture was captured by the high-speed camera. The test rig consisted of a pressure manometer, series of mirrors, pneumatic airline, pressure regulator and high-speed camera. When fully connected to the test rig, the silicone rubber model is constrained from movement at the proximal neck region, with the inside of each model dusted with calcium carbonate to ease visualisation of the rupture. The internal pressure was increased so that the rupture of the model occurred within 240s of testing, in accordance with the standards BS ISO 1402 for burst pressure tests. Air pressure readings were also recorded in the video image for analysis post-rupture. The test set-up as viewed through the high-speed camera is shown in Figure 29. All silicone rubber models were inflated until failure with each test recorded using the high-speed camera. Significance of rupture pressures and geometrical parameters were analysed using a Spearman's Rho correlation test in SPSS 15.

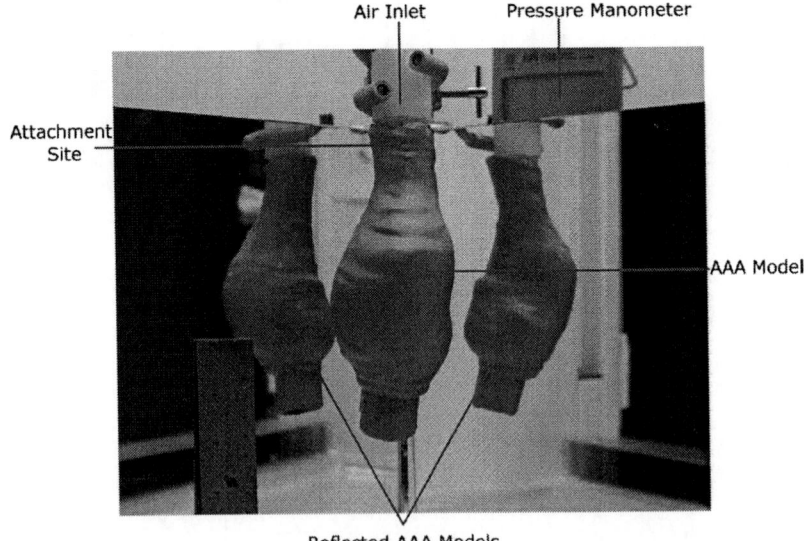

Figure 29: View through high-speed camera of test rig. Mirrors allow 360° of model to be captured. Model is constrained from movement proximally and distally. Pressure is continuously monitored with the manometer, while the model is inflated until rupture.

The results of the experimental rupture tests revealed a large range of burst pressures for the 16 unmixed AAA models as shown in Table 7. On average, the AAA models created using the weaker silicone rubber (Sylgard 170) ruptured at lower pressures than those made using the stronger silicone type (Sylgard 160). Sylgard 160 models ruptured at a mean ± SD pressure of 650.6 ± 195.1 mmHg (range = 381.4 – 985 mmHg), whereas the weaker Sylgard 170 ruptured at a mean ± SD pressure of 410.7 ± 159.9 mmHg (range = 252.2 – 714 mmHg). All realistic AAA geometries ruptured at regions of inflection. Only the Sylgard 160 models of Patient 1 ruptured at regions near the maximum diameter, although these rupture locations experienced localised inflection as there was a sharp change in curvature over a very short length. The location of rupture in other models varied. A typical sequence of events can be seen in Figure 30, showing the frames immediately prior to rupture, through to the point of complete failure. Case shown here is Patient 4 Sylgard 160 Model 1. The model in the centre of each image in Figure 30 is the original model, with the reflected views to either side. Table 8 shows the results for the mixed material models shown in Figure 28. The colour intensities recorded at the site of rupture correlates to a specific material type in Section 5.3.1. From the results to date, mixed AAA models appear to rupture at regions of lower UTS and also at regions of inflection. Interestingly, the ideal banded model ruptured below the AAA sac and not at the inflection zones or at the material intersection. The inflection zones in this case were made of the stronger Sylgard 160, with the model rupturing at a region of Sylgard 170.

Table 7. Rupture pressures and wall thickness at the site of rupture for each AAA case

		Sylgard 160			Sylgard 170	
	Model	Rupture Pressure (Mmhg)	Wall Thickness (Mm)	Model	Rupture Pressure (Mmhg)	Wall Thickness (Mm)
Patient 1	1	381.4	1.84	1	283.5	1.51
	2	985	2.03	2	309.8	1.7
Patient 2	1	909.8	1.41	1	459.3	1.41
	2	444.8	1.24	2	386.4	1.97
Patient 3	1	588.4	2.09	1	349.8	1.21
	2	629.8	1.78	2	252.2	1.57
Patient 4	1	736.9	2.34	1	320.2	2.1
	2	468	2.09	2	358.2	2.11

Table 8. Colour intensity results at the site of rupture for each model, the corresponding silicone type from previous work and the rupture pressure of each model

Model	ΔE	Corresponding Silicone Type	Rupture Pressure (mmHg)
Ideal 1	21.76	170	440
Ideal 2	26.05	70:30	395
Ideal 3	38.37	20:80	703
Ideal 4	25.67	80:20	703
Patient 1 Mixed	23.90	170	508

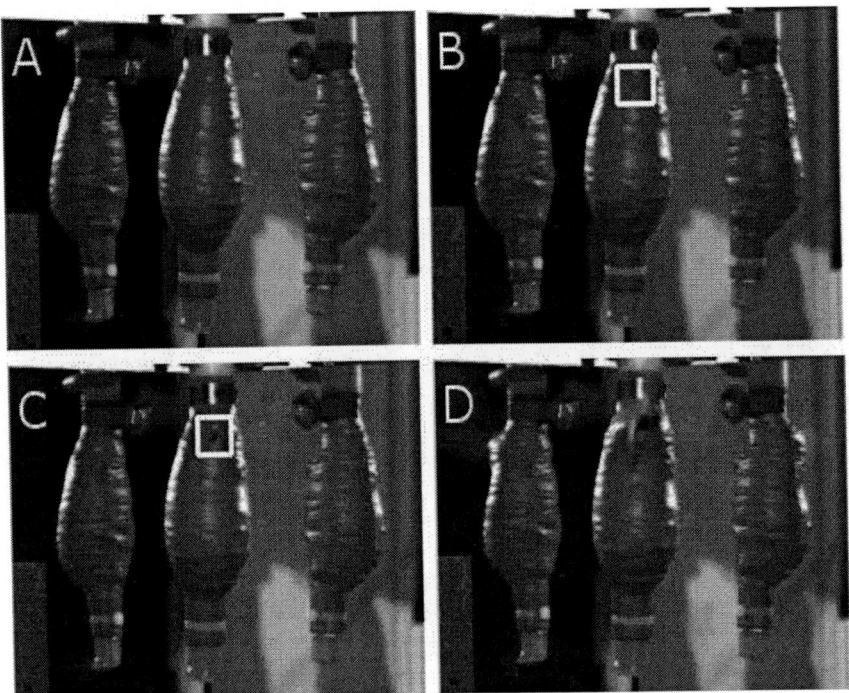

Figure 30. Typical sequence of events of rupture test. *(A)* Model is inflected with air, *(B)* silicone rubber fails (highlighted in figure), *(C)* tear develops (highlighted in figure) until *(D)* AAA model completely fails.

To correlate experimental and numerical results, the experiments were reproduced in the finite element solver ABAQUS v6.7. 3D reconstructions of the silicone models were used in these analyses and were reconstructed from

CT images taken of each experimental model. Constraints were placed at the proximal and distal regions of each model and a uniform static air pressure was applied to the internal surface of each model. For each numerical simulation, the average rupture pressure of that material was used as the loading condition. The Gaussian surface curvature was also determined for each AAA geometry using ProEngineer Wildfire 3.0. Surface curvature revealed complex distributions of surface curvature, which has been correlated to complex stress distributions by Sacks et al. [1999]. As shown in Figure 31 using one case as an example, the experimental sites of rupture agreed well with the numerically predicted regions of elevated wall stress and the Gaussian surface curvature. A similar trend was observed for all cases examined. Figure 32 compares the numerically predicted wall stress on the anterior region of the AAA with the isochromatic fringes obtained in Section 5.2 using the photoelastic method. The qualitative agreement between the computational and experimental studies can be seen. As with the numerical model, the photoelastic method resulted in a high stress region on the proximal anterior wall, which also proved to be the rupture site for this particular geometry.

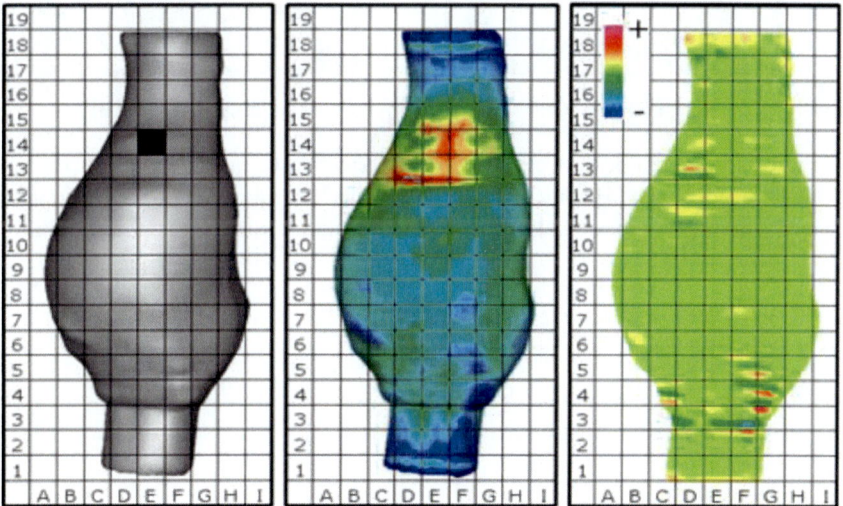

Figure 31. Comparison of experimental *(left)*, FEA *(centre)* and Gaussian surface curvature *(right)*. In the experimental results image the black mark indicates rupture site. In the FEA results image, red indicates high stress, and in the Gaussian surface curvature results, yellow/red regions indicate inflection points. Based on the three images in can be concluded that the inflection points encompass a region of high stress where the experimental model ruptured.

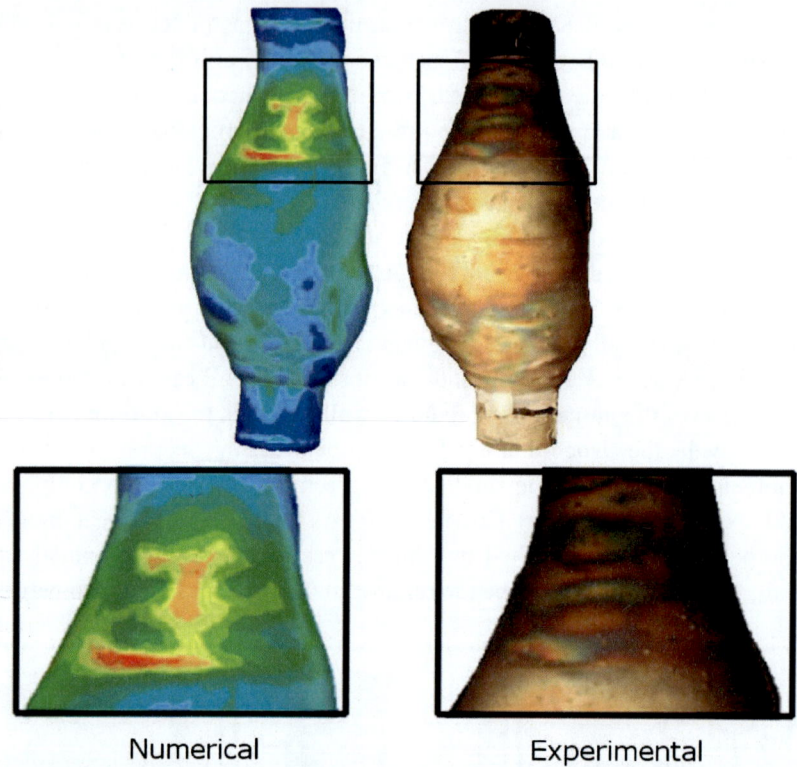

Figure 32. Comparison between FEA and the photoelastic method for a patient-specific AAA under 120 mmHg internal pressure. Model is shown from the anterior view. Good qualitative agreement was observed between the two methods.

Chapter 6

CONCLUSION

Throughout this chapter several approaches to AAA assessment and rupture potential have been explored, with some new insights and tools also reported. In contrast to many of the published findings available in the literature indicating the ineffective nature of diameter to accurately determine an AAAs rupture potential, diameter remains the key criterion in the decision-making process of the clinician. Over the past number of years, advancements in 3D imaging have allowed new techniques to be applied to AAA assessment, with 3D reconstruction of the diseased vessels now common practice. It is widely believed that alternative methods and factors should be included in the decision to surgically repair, with several approaches described and referenced in this chapter.

In order to compliment the advancements in 3D imaging and the use of this tool to aid AAA assessment, it is believed that improvements in numerical models may yield interesting results [Watton et al., 2004; Volokh and Vorp, 2008; Humphrey and Taylor, 2008]. It has been suggested that the incorporation of growth and remodelling factors into numerical models may also provide further insights in to the possibility of AAA rupture [Humphrey and Taylor, 2008]. Alongside improvements in numerical modelling, experimental tools and techniques can also be improved. By imaging the experimental model, for example using computed tomography, prior to testing allows exact numerical reconstructions to be generated, which greatly facilitates numerical validation of experiments.

"To operate or not to operate?" still remains a the key clinical question that is predominantly answered with the maximum diameter, yet, as portrayed throughout this book chapter and in the published literature, the diameter

criterion alone may not be adequate to comprehensively determine the severity of patient-specific AAAs. It is clear that 3D reconstructions of AAAs not only compliment traditional 2D images but also provide the basis for a range of alternative assessment tools such as those described throughout this chapter. These alternative tools can be used alongside the maximum diameter criterion and will improve the current trend in AAA assessment. There is a clear need to implement alternative factors in the clinical decision-making process and the many applications of 3D reconstructions reported in this chapter may be beneficial in the future of AAA assessment.

ACKNOWLEDGMENTS

The authors would like to acknowledge (i) the Irish Research Council for Science Engineering and Technology (IRCSET) and (ii) Grant No. RO1-HL-060670 from the United States Heart Lung and Blood Institute for funding this work. We would also like to thank Prof. David A. Vorp from the University of Pittsburgh for his help and guidance over the past number of years with our AAA research. Finally, the authors would like to thank the Centre for Applied Biomedical Engineering (CABER) in the University of Limerick and the HSE Midwestern Regional Hospital for all the support.

REFERENCES

Bosch, J.L., Lester, J.S., McMahon, P.M., Beinfeld, M.T. Halpern, E.F., Kaufman, J.A., Brewster, D.C., Gazelle, G.S. (2001) Hospital costs for elective endovascular and surgical repairs of infrarenal abdominal aortic aneurysms. *Radiology*, 220(2), 492-497.

Brosnan, M., Collins, C.G., Moneley, D.S., Kelly, C.J., Leahy, A.L. (2009) Making the case for cardiovascular screening in Irish males: Detection of abdominal aortic aneurysms, and assessment of cardiovascular risk factors. *European Journal of Vascular and Endovascular Surgery*, 37, 300-304.

Cabral, B., Cam N., Foran, J. (1994) Accelerated volume rendering and tomographic reconstruction using texture mapping hardware, *Proceedings 1994 ACM/IEEE Symposium on Volume Visualisation*, 91-97.

Calhoun, P.S., Kuszyk, B.S., Heath, D.G., Carley, J.C., Fishman, E.K. (1999) Three-dimensional volume rendering of spiral CT data: Theory and method, *Radiographics*, 19, 745-764.

Callanan, A., Morris, L.G., McGloughlin, T.M. (2004) Numerical and experimental analysis of an idealised abdominal aortic aneurysm. *European Society of Biomechanics, S-Hertogenbosch, Netherlands*.

Chong CK, How TV. (2004) Flow patterns in an endovascular stent-graft for abdominal aortic aneurysm repair. *Journal of Biomechanics*, 37, 89-97.

Conway, K.P., Byrne, J., Townsend, M., Lane, I.F. (2001) Prognosis of patients turned down for conventional abdominal aortic aneurysm repair in the endovascular and sonographic era: Szilagyi revisted? *Journal of Vascular Surgery*, 33, 752-757.

Corbett, T.J., Callanan, A., Morris, L.G., Doyle, B.J., Grace, P.A., Kavanagh, E.G. McGloughlin, T.M. (2008) A review of the in vivo and in vitro biomechanical behaviour and performance of postoperative abdominal aortic aneurysms and implanted stent-grafts. *Journal of Endovascular Therapy*, 15, 468-464.

Creagh, D., Neilson, S., Collins, A., Colwell, N., Hinchion, R., Drew, C., O'Halloran, D., Perry, I.J. (2002) Established cardiovascular disease and CVD risk factors in a primary care population of middle-aged Irish men and women. *Irish Medical Journal*, 95(10), 298-301.

Cronenwett, J.L., Murphy, T.F., Zelenock, G.B., Whitehouse Jr., W.M., Lindenauer, S.M., Graham, L.M., Quint, L.E., Silver, T.M., Stanley, J.C. (1985) Actuarial analysis of variables associated with rupture of small abdominal aortic aneurysms. *Surgery*, 98, 472-483.

Darling, R.C., Messina, C.R., Brewster, D.C., Ottinger, L.W. (1977) Autopsy study of unoperated abdominal aortic aneurysms. The case for early resection. *Circulation*, 56(2), 161-164.

Department of Health and Children: Dublin. (1999) Building Healthier Hearts: The report of the cardiovascular health strategy group.

Di Martino, E.S., Guadagni, G., Fumero, A., Ballerini, G., Spirito, R., Biglioli, P, Redaelli, A. (2001) Fluid-structure interaction within realistic 3D models of aneurysmatic aorta as a guidance to assess the risk of rupture of the aneurysm. *Medical Engineering and Physics*, 23, 647-655.

Doyle, B.J., Callanan, A., McGloughlin, T.M. (2007) A comparison of modelling techniques for computing wall stress in abdominal aortic aneurysms. *Biomedical Engineering Online*, 6, 38.

Doyle, B.J., Morris, L.G., Callanan, A., Kelly, P., Vorp, D.A., McGloughlin, T.M. (2008a) 3D reconstruction and manufacture of real abdominal aortic aneurysms: From CT scan to silicone model. *Journal of Biomechanical Engineering*, 130, 034501.

Doyle, B.J., Callanan, A., Corbett, T.J., Cloonan, A.J., O'Donnell, M.R., Vorp, D.A., McGloughlin, T.M. (2008b) The use of silicone to model abdominal aortic aneurysm behaviour. *Society of Plastics Engineers, SPE European Conference on Medical Polymers*, 115-120.

Doyle, B.J., Callanan, A., Burke, P.E., Grace, P.A., Walsh, M.T., Vorp, D.A., McGloughlin, T.M. (2009a) Vessel asymmetry as an additional tool in the assessment of abdominal aortic aneurysms. *Journal of Vascular Surgery*, 49, 443-454.

Doyle, B.J., Callanan, A., Walsh, M.T., Grace, P.A., McGloughlin, T.M. (2009b) A finite element analysis rupture index (FEARI) as an additional tool for abdominal aortic aneurysm rupture prediction. *Vascular Disease Prevention*, 6, 114-121.

Doyle, B.J., Grace, P.A. Kavanagh, E.G., Burke, P.E. Wallis, F., Walsh, M.T., McGloughlin, T.M. (2009c) Improved assessment and treatment of abdominal aortic aneurysms: The use of 3D reconstructions as a surgical guidance tool in endovascular repair. *Irish Journal of Medical Science*, 178, 321–328.

Doyle, B.J., Corbett, T.J., Callanan, A., Walsh, M.T., Vorp, D.A., McGloughlin, T.M. (2009d) An experimental and numerical comparison of the rupture locations of an abdominal aortic aneurysm. *Journal of Endovascular Therapy*, 16, 322-335.

Doyle, B.J., Corbett, T.J., Cloonan, A.J., O'Donnell, M.R., Walsh, M.T., Vorp, D.A., McGloughlin, T.M. (2009e) Experimental Modelling of Abdominal Aortic Aneurysms: Novel Applications of Silicone Rubbers. *Medical Engineering and Physics*, in press, doi:10.1016/j.medengphy.2009.06.002.

Egelhoff, C.J., Buduig, R.S., Elger D.F., Khraishi, T.A., Johansen K.H. (1999) Model studies of the flow in abdominal aortic aneurysms during resting and exercise conditions. *Journal of Biomechanics*, 32, 1319-1329.

Ernst, C.B. (1993) Abdominal aortic aneurysm. *The New England Journal of Medicine*, 328(16), 1167-1172.

EVAR Trial Participants. (2004) Comparison of endovascular aneurysm repair with open repair in patients with abdominal aortic aneurysm (EVAR trial 1), 30-day operative mortality results: randomised controlled trial. *The Lancet*, 364, 843-848.

EVAR Trial Participants (2005a) Endovascular aneurysm repair versus open repair in patients with abdominal aortic aneurysm (EVAR Trial 1): randomised controlled trial. *The Lancet*, 365, 2179-2186.

EVAR Trial Participants (2005b) Endovascular aneurysm repair and outcome in patients unfit for open repair of abdominal aortic aneurysm (EVAR Trail 2): randomised controlled trial. *The Lancet*, 365(9578), 2187-2192.

Fraunhofer SCAI: MpCCI Documentation. *Sankt Augustin, Germany;* 2008

Fillinger, M.F., Marra, S.P., Raghavan, M.L., Kennedy, F.E. (2003) Prediction of rupture risk in abdominal aortic aneurysm during observation: wall stress versus diameter. *Journal of Vascular Surgery*, 37, 724-732.

Fillinger, M.F., Raghavan, M.L., Marra, S.P., Cronenwett, J.L., Kennedy, F.E. (2002) In vivo analysis of mechanical wall stress and abdominal aortic aneurysm rupture risk. *Journal of Vascular Surgery*, 36, 589-597.

Flora, H.S., Talei-Faz, B., Ansell, L., Chaloner, E.J., Sweeny, A., Grass, A., Adiseshiah, M. (2002) Aneurysm wall stress and tendency to rupture are features of physical wall properties: an experimental study. *Journal of Endovascular Therapy*, 9(5), 665-675.

Garcia-Madrid, C., Josa, M., Riambau, V., Mestresa, C.A., Muntanab, J., Muleta, J. (2004) Endovascular versus open surgical repair of abdominal aortic aneurysm: a comparison of early and intermediate results in patients suitable for both techniques. *Journal of Endovascular Therapy*, 28(4), 365-372.

Giannoglu, G., Giannakoulas, G., Soulis, J., Chatzizisis, Y., Perdikides, T., Melas, N., Parcharidis, G., Louridas, G. (2006) Predicting the risk of rupture of abdominal aortic aneurysms by utilizing various geometrical parameters: Revisiting the diameter criterion. *Angiology*, 57(4), 487-494.

Glimaker, H., Holmberg, L., Elvin, A., Nybacka, O., Almgren, B., Bjorck, C.G., Eriksson, I. (1991) Natural history of patients with abdominal aortic aneurysm. *European Journal of Vascular Surgery*, 5, 125-130.

Goueffic, Y., Becquemin, J.P., Desgranges, P., Kobeiter, H. (2005) Midterm survival after endovascular versus open repair of infrarenal aortic aneurysms. *Journal of Endovascular Therapy*, 12(1), 47-57.

Hirose, Y., Takamiya, M. (1998) Growth curve of ruptured aortic aneurysm. *Journal of Cardiovascular Surgery*, 39, 9-13.

Howell, B.A., Kim, T., Cheer, A. Dwyer, H., Saloner, D., Chuter, T.A. (2007) Computational fluid dynamics within bifurcated abdominal aortic stent-grafts. *Journal of Endovascular Therapy*, 14, 138-143.

Hua, J., Mower, W.R. (2001) Simple geometric characteristics fail to reliably predict abdominal aortic aneurysm wall stress. *Journal of Vascular Surgery*, 34, 308-315.

Humphrey, J.D., Taylor, C.A. (2008) Intracranial and abdominal aortic aneurysms: Similarities, differences, and need for a new computational class. *Annual Review of Biomedical Engineering*, 10, 221-246.

Inzoli, F., Boschetti, F., Zappa, M., Longo, T., Fumero, R. (1993) Biomechanical factors in abdominal aortic aneurysm rupture. *European Journal of Vascular Surgery*, 7, 667-674.

Jacobowitz, G.R., Lee, A.M., Riles, T.S. (1999) Immediate and late explantation of endovascular aortic grafts: the EndoVascular Technologies experience. *Journal of Vascular Surgery*, 29, 309-316.

Kamineni, R. and Heuser, R. (2004) Abdominal aortic aneurysm: a review of endoluminal treatment. *Journal of Interventional Cardiology*, 17, 437-445.

Kleinstreuer, C. and Li, Z. (2006) Analysis and computer program for rupture-risk prediction of abdominal aortic aneurysms. *Biomedical Engineering Online*, 5, 19.

Laheij, R., van Marrewijk, C., Buth, J. (2001) Progress report on the procedural and follow up results of 3413 patients who received stent graft treatment for infrarenal aortic aneurysms for a period of 6 years. *EUROSTAR Data Registry Centre*.

Lederle, F.A., Johnson, G.R., Wilson, S.E., Ballard, D.J., Jordan Jr., W.D., Blebea, J., Littooy, F.N., Freischlag, J.A., Bandyk, D., Rapp, J.H., Salam, A.A. (2002) Rupture rate of large abdominal aortic aneurysms in patients refusing or unfit for elective repair. *Journal of the American Medical Association*, 287, 2968-2972.

Leung, J.H., Wright, A.R., Cheshire, N., Crane, J., Thom, S.A., Hughes, A.D., Xu, Y. (2006) Fluid structure interaction of patient specific abdominal aortic aneurysms: a comparison with solid stress models. *Biomedical Engineering Online*, 5, 33.

Li, Z. and Kleinstreuer, C. (2005a) Blood flow and structure interactions in stented abdominal aortic aneurysm model. *Medical Engineering and Physics*, 27, 369-382.

Li, Z. and Kleinstreuer, C. (2005b) A new wall stress equation for aneurysm-rupture. *Annals of Biomedical Engineering*, 33(2), 209-213.

Lorensen, W.E. and H.E. Cline, H.E. (1987) Marching Cubes: A high resolution 3D surface construction algorithm, *Computer Graphics*, 21(4), 163-169.

Loth, F., Jones, S.A., Giddens, D.P., Bassiouny, H.S., Glagov, S., Zarins, C.K. (1997) Measurements of velocity and wall shear stress inside a ptfe vascular graft model under steady flow conditions. *Journal of Biomechanical Engineering*, 119(2), 187-194.

Mills, C., Gabe, I., Gault, J., Mason, D., Ross, J. (1970) Pressure-flow relationships and vascular impedance in man. *Cardiovascular Research*, 4, 405-417

Molony, D.S., Callanan, A., Morris, L.G., Doyle, B.J., Walsh, M.T., McGloughlin, T.M. (2008) Geometrical enhancements for abdominal aortic stent-grafts. *Journal of Endovascular Therapy*, 15, 518-529.

Morris, L., Delassus, P., Walsh, M., McGloughlin, T. (2004a) A mathematical model to predict in vivo pulsatile drag forces acting on bifurcated stent grafts used in endovascular treatment of abdominal aortic aneurysms (AAA). *Journal of Biomechanics*, 37, 1087-1095.

Morris, L., O'Donnell, P., Delassus, P., McGloughlin, T. (2004b) Experimental assessment of stress patterns in abdominal aortic aneurysms using the photoelastic method. *Strain*, 40, 165-172.

Morris, L., Delassus, P., Grace, P., Wallis, F., Walsh, M., McGloughlin, T. (2006a) Effects of flat, parabolic and realistic steady flow inlet profiles on idealised and realistic stent graft fits through abdominal aortic aneurysm (AAA). *Medical Engineering and Physics*, 28, 19-26.

Morris, L., McGloughlin, T., Dellasus, P., Walsh, M., O'Brien, T., Callanan, A. (2006b) A vascular graft. International Patent WO 2006/103641 A1.

Mower, W.R., Quinones, W.J., Gambhir, S.S. (1997) Effect of intraluminal thrombus on abdominal aortic aneurysm wall stress. *Journal of Vascular Surgery*, 26, 602-608.

Mullins, L. (1969) Softening of rubber by deformation. Rubber Chemistry and Technology, 42, 339-62.

National Health Service (2009) National Screening Program for Abdominal Aortic Aneurysm [online] available: http://aaa.screening.nhs.uk [accessed 9 Feb 2009].

Nicholls, S.C., Gardner, J.B., Meissner, M.H., Johansen, H.K. (1998) Rupture in small abdominal aortic aneurysms. *Journal of Vascular Surgery*, 28, 884-888.

O'Brien, T., Morris, L., O'Donnell, M., Walsh, M., McGloughlin, T. (2005) Injection-moulded models of major and minor arteries: The variability of model wall thickness owing to casting technique. *Proceedings of the International Mechanical Engineers, Part H: Journal of Engineering in Medicine*, 219.

O'Brien, T., Morris, L., McGloughlin, T. (2008) Evidence suggests rigid aortic graft increase systolic blood pressure: results of a preliminary study. *Medical Engineering and Physics*, 30, 109-115.

Papaharilaou, Y., Ekaterinaris, J.A., Manoussaki, E., Katsamouris, A.N. (2007) A decoupled fluid structure approach for estimating wall stress in abdominal aortic aneurysms. *Journal of Biomechanics*, 40, 367-377.

Parodi, J.C., Palmaz, J.C., Barone, H.D. (1991) Transfemoral intraluminal graft implantation for treatment of abdominal aortic aneurysms. *Annals of Vascular Surgery*, 5, 491-499.

Quill, D.S., Colgan, M.P., Sumner, D.S. (1989) Ultrasonic screening for the detection of abdominal aortic aneurysms. *Surgical Clinics of North America*, 69, 713-720.

Raghavan, M.L., Kratzberg, J., de Tolosa, E.M.C., Hanaoka, M.M., Walter, P., da Silva, E.S. (2006) Regional distribution of wall thickness and failure properties of human abdominal aortic aneurysm. *Journal of Biomechanics*, 39(16), 3010-6.

Raghavan, M.L. and Vorp, D.A. (2000) Toward a biomechanical tool to evaluate rupture potential of abdominal aortic aneurysm: identification of a finite strain constitutive model and evaluation of its applicability. *Journal of Vascular Surgery*, 33, 475-482.

Raghavan, M.L., Vorp, D.A., Federle, M.P., Makaroun, M.S., Webster, M.W. (2000) Wall stress distribution on three-dimensionally reconstructed models of human abdominal aortic aneurysm. *Journal of Vascular Surgery*, 31, 760-769.

Raghavan, M.L., Webster, M.W., Vorp, D.A. (1996) Ex vivo biomechanical behaviour of abdominal aortic aneurysm: assessment using a new mathematical model. *Annals of Biomedical Engineering*, 24, 573-582.

Rissland, P., Alemu, Y., Einav, S., Ricotta, J., Bluestein, D. (2009) Abdominal aortic aneurysm risk of rupture: Patient-specific FSI simulations using anisotropic model. *Journal of Biomechanical Engineering*, 131, 031001.

Sacks, M.S., Vorp, D.A., Raghavan, M.L., Federle, M.P., Webster, M.W. (1999) In vivo three-dimensional surface geometry of abdominal aortic aneurysms. *Annals of Biomedical Engineering*, 27(4), 469-479.

Sakalihasan, N., Limet, R., Defawe, O.D. (2005) Abdominal aortic aneurysm. *The Lancet*, 365(9470), 1577-89.

Sayers, R.D. (2002) Aortic aneurysms, inflammatory pathways and nitric oxide. *Annals of the Royal College of Surgeons England*, 84(4), 239-246.

Scotti, C.M., Finol, E.A. (2007) Compliant biomechanics of abdominal aortic aneurysms: a fluid-structure interaction study. *Computers and Structures*. 85, 1097-1113.

Scotti, C.M., Shkolnik, A.D., Muluk, S.C., Finol, E. (2005) Fluid-structure interaction in abdominal aortic aneurysms: effect of asymmetry and wall thickness. *Biomedical Engineering Online*, 4, 64.

Seong, J., Sadasivan, C., Onizuka, M., Gounis, M.J., Christian, F., Miskolczi, L., Wakhloo, A.K., Lieber B.B. (2005) Morphology of elastase-induced cerebral aneurysm model in rabbit and rapid prototyping of elastomeric transparent replicas. *Biorheology*, 42(5), 345-361.

Shipkowitz, T., Rodgers, V., Frazin, L., Chandran, C.B. (1998) Numerical study on the effect of steady axial flow development in the human aorta on local shear stresses in abdominal aortic branches. *Journal of Biomechanics*, 31, 995-1007.

Speelman, L., Bohra, A., Bosboom, E.M.H., Schurink, G.W.H., van de Vosse, F.N., Makaroun, M.S., Vorp, D.A. (2007) Effects of wall calcifications in patient-specific wall stress analyses of abdominal aortic aneurysms. *Journal of Biomechanical Engineering*, 129, 1-5.

Stenbaek, J., Kalin, B., Swedenborg, J. (2000) Growth of thrombus may be a better predictor of rupture than diameter in patients with abdominal aortic aneurysms. *European Journal of Vascular and Endovascular Surgery*, 20, 466-469.

Thubrikar, M.J., Labrosse, M., Robicsek, F., Al-Soudi, J., Fowler, B. (2001a) Mechanical properties of abdominal aortic aneurysm wall. *Journal of Medical Engineering and Technology*, 25(4), 133-142.

Thubrikar, M.J., Al-Soudi, J., Robicsek, F. (2001b) Wall stress studies of abdominal aortic aneurysm in a clinical model. *Annals of Vascular Surgery*, 15, 355-366.

Truijers, M., Pol, J.A., SchultzeKool, L.J., van Sterkenburg, S.M., Fillinger, M.F., Blankensteijn, J.D. (2007) Wall stress analysis in small asymptomatic, symptomatic and ruptured abdominal aortic aneurysms. *European Journal of Vascular and Endovascular Surgery*, 33, 401-407.

United States Preventative Services Task Force (USPSTF). (2005) Screening for abdominal aortic aneurysm: Recommendation statement. *Annals of Internal Medicine*, 142(3), 198-202.

Vande Geest, J.P., Wang, D.H.J., Wisniewski, S.R., Makaroun, M.S., Vorp, D.A (2006a) Towards a non-invasive method for determination of patient-specific wall strength distribution in abdominal aortic aneurysms. *Annals of Biomedical Engineering*, 34(7), 1098-1106.

Vande Geest, J.P., Di Martino, E.S., Bohra, A., Makaroun, M.S., Vorp, D.A. (2006b) A biomechanics-based rupture potential index for abdominal aortic aneurysm risk assessment. *Annals of the New York Academy of Science*, 1085, 11-21.

Venkatasubramaniam, A.K., Fagan, M.J., Mehta, T., Mylankal, K.J., Ray, B., Kuhan, G., Chetter, I.C., McCollum, P.T. (2004) A comparative study of aortic wall stress using finite element analysis for ruptured and non-ruptured abdominal aortic aneurysms. *European Journal of Vascular and Endovascular Surgery*, 28, 168-176.

Vierendeels, J.D., Lanoye, L., Degroote, J., Verdonck, P. (2007) Implicit coupling of partitioned fluid-structure interaction problems with reduce order models. *Computers and Structures*, 85, 970-976

Vogel, T.R., Nackman, G.B., Crowley, J.G., Bueno, M.M., Banavage, A., Odroniec, K., Brevetti, L.S., Ciocca, R.G., Graham, A.M. (2005) Factors impacting functional health and resource utilisation following abdominal aortic aneurysm repair by open and endovascular techniques. *Annals of Vascular Surgery*, 19, 641-647.

Volokh, K.Y. and Vorp, D.A. (2008) A model of growth and rupture of abdominal aortic aneurysm. *Journal of Biomechanics*, 41(5), 1015-21.

Vorp, D.A. (2007) Biomechanics of abdominal aortic aneurysm. *Journal of Biomechanics*, 40(9), 1887-1902.

Vorp, D.A., Raghavan, M.L., Webster, M.W. (1998) Mechanical wall stress in abdominal aortic aneurysm: influence of diameter and asymmetry. *Journal of Vascular Surgery*, 27(4), 632-639.

Vorp, D.A., Vande Geest, J. (2005) Biomechanical determinants of abdominal aortic aneurysm rupture. *Arteriosclerosis, Thrombosis and Vascular Biology*, 25, 1558-1566.

Wang, D.H.J., Makaroun, M.S., Webster, M.W., Vorp, D.A. (2002) Effect of intraluminal thrombus on wall stress in patient-specific models of abdominal aortic aneurysm. *Journal of Vascular Surgery*, 36, 598-604.

Wang, D.H.J., Makaroun, M., Webster, M.W., Vorp, D.A. (2001) Mechanical properties and microstructure of intraluminal thrombus from abdominal aortic aneury

Watton, P., Hill, N., Heil, M. (2004) A mathematical model for the growth of the abdominal aortic aneurysm. *Biomechanics and Modelling in Mechanobiology*, 3(2), 98-113.

Webb, S. (1988) *The Physics of medical imaging. 1st ed.* London: Institute of Physics Publishing.

INDEX

A

accuracy, 55, 56
acetone, 54
ACM, 81
age, 1, 3, 4, 18, 29, 43
agent, 54
aiding, 37
air, 57, 69, 73
algorithm, 12, 46, 87
alternative, xiii, 24, 32, 77, 78
aluminium, 51, 52
anatomy, 8
angina, 6
aorta, xii, 1, 3, 7, 19, 21, 22, 23, 25, 30, 31, 38, 39, 44, 64, 82, 91
aortic aneurysm, xii, 1, 2, 19, 20, 81, 82, 83, 84, 85, 86, 87, 88, 89, 90, 91, 92, 93
appendicitis, 8
application, 8, 25, 45, 59
arterial vessels, 50
arteries, 1, 18, 22, 25, 31, 44, 50, 55, 88
artery, 7, 18, 30, 32, 46
assessment, xii, xiii, xiv, 5, 30, 37, 44, 77, 78, 81, 83, 88, 90
assessment tools, 78
asymmetry, 6, 17, 29, 31, 32, 34, 36, 37, 43, 83, 90, 93
asymptomatic, 3, 91

attachment, 46, 51, 64
autopsy, 5
averaging, 40

B

bell, 59, 61
benefits, xiii, 24, 28, 45
bifurcation, 22, 24, 26, 30, 31, 54
bifurcation point, 24
biomechanics, 16, 17, 35, 44, 90, 92
blocks, 51
blood flow, 7, 23, 48
blood pressure, 24, 31, 39, 46
blood vessels, 8
boundary conditions, 30, 38, 46, 61
bowel, 8
bowel obstruction, 8

C

CAD, 17, 49, 51, 53, 56
calcium, 70
calcium carbonate, 70
calibration, 57, 58, 60, 61, 62
cardiovascular disease, 1, 8, 82
cardiovascular risk, 81
case study, 49
cast, 5, 50
casting, 50, 54, 89
cerebral aneurysm, 90
cerebral arteries, 8

CFD, 15, 23, 24, 27
chronic obstructive pulmonary disease, 2
clinician, 9, 17, 18, 19, 20, 21, 23, 33, 36, 42, 44, 49, 77
codes, 45, 51
community, 21
complexity, 51
complications, 7, 18, 21, 22, 48, 49
computation, 29
computational fluid dynamics, xii, 15
computed tomography, 4, 8, 77
computer graphics, 12
computer technology, 49
computing, 12, 39, 83
concentration, 60, 65
congestive heart failure, 6
connective tissue, 2
constraints, 30
construction, 12, 87
control, 28, 29, 46, 51
convex, 67
correlation, 34, 40, 56, 60, 67, 70
correlations, 34, 60
cost-effective, 4, 24
costs, 81
coupling, 45, 46, 92
cross-sectional, 9
curing, 55
CVD, 82
cycles, 59

D

data set, 13, 49
death, 3
deaths, 1, 3, 4
decision making, 36, 42
decision-making process, xiii, 77, 78
defects, 55
definition, 39
deformation, 38, 66, 88
degradation, 2
density, 25, 46
detection, 4, 12, 33, 89
diet, 4
dilation, 1, 2, 36

discrete data, 12
disorder, 2
displacement, 30, 65, 66
distraction, 50
distribution, 23, 41, 65, 69, 89, 92
diverticulitis, 8
durability, 7

E

elastomers, 59
elderly, 1, 3
Emergency Medical Services, v
encapsulated, 10
energy, 38, 61
energy density, 38
estimating, 89
exercise, 84
extraction, 12

F

fabric, 7
failure, 5, 37, 39, 58, 59, 70, 71, 89
family history, 2, 43
FEM, 5, 37, 38, 39, 40
females, 29
fibrin, 6
finite element method, 5, 65
fixation, 18
flow, 7, 17, 21, 22, 23, 24, 25, 46, 48, 50, 84, 87, 88, 91
flow rate, 46
fluid mechanics, 24
freedom, 46
funding, 79

G

gender, 2, 43
generation, 21, 44
geometrical parameters, 6, 41, 70, 85
gold, 7, 8
gold standard, 7, 8
grafts, 21, 22, 24, 25, 86, 88
growth, 6, 21, 77, 92, 93
guidance, 35, 79, 82, 83

H

health, 3, 8, 16, 82, 92
health problems, 3
heart, 6
height, 29
hemodynamics, 56
high resolution, 87
high-risk, 35
high-speed, 67, 69, 71
homogenous, 31, 38, 45, 58
hospital, 3
human, 7, 89, 91
hydrostatic pressure, 46
hypertension, 2

I

imaging, xii, xiii, 3, 6, 7, 16, 21, 29, 46, 77, 93
imaging techniques, 8
implementation, 3
in vitro, 15, 24, 82
in vivo, 30, 38, 58, 64, 82, 88
incidence, 3
inclusion, 43
incompressible, 24, 31, 38, 45
independence, 39, 66
indication, 59
inflammatory, 90
injection, 49, 64
insight, 62
institutions, 4
integration, 30
interaction, xii, 15, 45, 49, 82, 87, 90, 92
interactions, 87
intervention, 5, 6, 7, 21, 37, 44
invasive, 7
investigations, xi, 17, 53
ionic, 29
ionizing radiation, 8
isotropic, 31, 38, 45

L

lamina, 24
laminar, 24
language, 12
laser, 50
layering, 13, 53, 54
learning, 21
life expectancy, 7
lifestyle, 4
likelihood, xiii, 4, 17, 49
limitations, 22
linear, 31, 45, 60, 62
localised, 1, 71
location, 40, 42, 44, 50, 67, 71
lumen, 10, 18, 44, 46, 54
luminal, 39

M

magnetic, viii, xii, 8
magnetic resonance imaging, xii, 8
males, 4, 29, 81
manufacturer, 21
manufacturing, 17, 50, 53, 60
mapping, 13, 81
mathematics, 8
matrix, 12
measurement, 21, 33, 64, 65
measures, 31
medicine, 1
melt, 55
men, 3, 4, 82
microstructure, 93
middle-aged, 82
migration, xiii, 7, 22, 24, 49
mixing, 68, 69
morphology, 17, 21
mortality, 1, 3, 84
mortality rate, 1, 3
moulding, 49
movement, 64, 65, 70, 71
MRI, 8
myocardial infarction, 6

N

National Health Service, 4, 88
neck, 18, 24, 34, 47, 48, 64, 66, 70
nitric oxide, 90
nodes, 30, 45
non-invasive, 5, 8, 92
non-Newtonian fluid, 45
non-uniform, 30
normal, 1, 7, 8, 23
novel materials, 63
novelty, 24
numerical analysis, 5
numerical tool, 19, 23, 29, 49

O

obesity, 4
occlusion, 22
online, 88
operator, 12, 46
orientation, 37
oxide, 90

P

pancreatitis, 8
parabolic, 88
parameter, 33
pathways, 90
physiology, 8
platelets, 6
play, 37, 42
polynomial, 61
poor, 53
population, 3, 38, 46, 63, 82
postoperative, 82
preconditioning, 59
pregnant women, 8
premature death, 1
primary care, 82
production, 56
program, 4, 86
proteins, 6
prototyping, 50
pulse, 24, 25, 47

R

radiation, 8
radiologists, 33
random, 64, 65, 69
range, 8, 11, 18, 29, 40, 50, 58, 66, 71, 78
rapid prototyping, 91
reality, 36, 49, 53
regional, 40
registry, 87
relationship, 32, 37, 41, 58, 61, 62
remodelling, 77
renal, 6, 8, 18, 30, 31, 32, 39
replication, 56
resection, 82
resistance, 59
resolution, 8, 12, 87
returns, 23, 39
risk assessment, 92
risk factors, 2, 81, 82
risks, 4
rubber, 53, 54, 56, 58, 60, 70, 71, 73, 88

S

sample, 59, 60, 61
screening programs, 3
segmentation, 11, 12, 28
separation, 22
series, 30, 31, 33, 70
severity, 4, 15, 44, 78
shape, 9, 41
shear, 24, 27, 87, 91
simulation, 47, 73, 90
sites, xiii, 18, 74
skewness, 45
smoking, 2, 4, 43
smoothing, 15, 28, 29, 30
solidification, 55
spectrophotometer, 59, 65
spectrophotometry, 68
speed, 59, 67, 69, 71
standard deviation, 29, 41
standards, 70
statistics, 3

strain, 38, 57, 59, 61, 63, 64, 89
strains, 30
stroke, 7
surgeons, 21, 37
surgery, 5, 44
surgical intervention, 5, 6, 37, 44
survival, 85
systems, 49, 53
systolic blood pressure, 89
systolic pressure, 31, 39, 46, 48

T

temperature, 54
tensile, 6, 37, 39, 59, 60, 61, 63
tensile strength, 37, 61
therapy, 15
thoracic, 1, 19, 20
three-dimensional, 13, 89, 90
threshold, 12, 19, 29, 37
thrombosis, 21, 22
thrombus, 6, 44, 46, 88, 91, 93
time, 7, 37, 44, 48, 49
tissue, 2, 8, 37, 39, 40, 43

tobacco smoking, 2
transition, 24, 26
transparent, 91
trial, 84

U

ultrasonography, 3, 4, 8
ultrasound, 6, 8
uniform, 30, 55, 65, 73

V

variability, 88
variables, 39, 82
variance, 12
variation, 59, 67
velocity, 25, 26, 27, 46, 48, 87
vessels, 77
viscosity, 25, 46
visible, 29
vortex, 48, 49
women, 3, 4, 8, 82